Intermittent Fastin

Over 60 + Anti-Inflammatory Diet

Cookbook for Beginners

2 BOOKS IN 1

A Complete Guide for women to learn what happens after they turn 60, with Delicious and Simple Recipes to Reduce Inflammation and Boost Their Immune System.

By

MELINDA FRANCIS

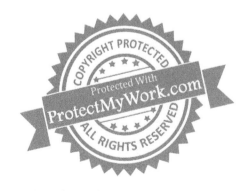

TABLE OF CONTENTS 2 BOOKS IN 1

Introduction..

Chapter 1: What Happens To A Women's Body After 60...**10**

1.1 Metabolism System of Women over 60..10

1.2 HGH Production Level in Women 11

1.3 Other Effects of Aging:...12

Chapter 2: What Is Intermittent Fasting?...**14**

2.1 Benefits of Intermittent Fasting for Women over 60's...15

2.2 The Truth about Intermittent Fasting...17

2.3 Why start Intermittent Fasting After the '60s...18

2.4 How is Intermittent Fasting Riskier for Women over 60?..18

Chapter 3: Types Of Intermittent Fasting..**23**

3.1 A weekly 24-hour Fast..23

3.2 12 hrs a day Fast...24

3.3 Fasting for 16 hrs...25

3.4 The Warrior Diet...26

3.5 Alternate Day Fasting...26

3.6 5:2 Method...27

3.7 Meal Skipping..28

Chapter 4: How to Start Intermittent Fasting?...**29**

4.1 Set Your Smart Goals..29

4.2 Deal with Hunger Pangs...30

4.3 Practice Portion Control..33

Chapter 5: Breakfast Recipes For Intermittent Fasting..**35**

5.1 Fat Burning Green Smoothie...35

5.2 Low Carb Pancakes..35

5.3 Keto Tumeric Milkshake...36

5.4 Breakfast Burritos..36

5.5 Fat-Burning Coconut Cookies...37

5.6 Spinach Frittata...37

5.7 Low-Calorie Porridge..38

Chapter 6: Lunch Recipes For Intermittent Fasting..**39**

6.1 Jars of Chicken Spring Rolls...39

6.2 Zucchini Noodle Casserole...39

6.3 Fish Tacos..40

6.4 Lemon Green Beans..41

6.5 Eggplant Parmesan Panini..41

6.6 Paleo Chicken Stew..42

6.7 Chicken Salad with Walnuts and Grapes...43

Chapter 7: Dinner Recipes For Intermittent Fasting..44

7.1 Honey Sesame Salmon..44

7.2 Chicken with Cauliflower Rice Casserole..44

7.3 Lentil and Vegetable Curry..45

7.4 Honey Garlic Shrimp..46

7.5 Turkey Meatball and Kale Soup..46

7.6 Chicken Provolone...47

7.7 Spaghetti Diablo with Shrimp...47

Chapter 8: Dessert Recipes For Intermittent Fasting...49

8.1 Citrus Dark Chocolate Mousse..49

8.2 Peanut Butter Cookies...49

8.3 Fruit Salad...50

8.1 Grapefruit Meringue Nests with Mixed Berries..51

8.5 Mango and Passionfruit Roulade..51

8.6 Strawberry-Chocolate Greek Yogurt..52

8.7 Almond Butter Chocolate Chip Cookies...52

Conclusion...54

Introduction..55

CHAPTER 1: What exactly is meant by the term "anti-inflammatory diet"?..........56

CHAPTER 2: Anti-inflammatory Breakfast Recipes...59

2.1 Chia Seed and Milk Pudding..59

2.2 Scrambled Eggs with Turmeric...60

2.3 Protein-Rich Turmeric Donuts..60

2.4 Cranberry and Sweet Potato Bars..61

2.5 Nutty Choco-Nana Pancakes..61

2.6 Blueberry Avocado Chocolate Muffins...62

2.7 Tropical Smoothie Container..62

2.8 Smoked Salmon in Scrambled Eggs...63

2.9 Spinach and Potatoes with Smoked Salmon...63

2.10 Eggs in a Mushroom and Bacon...64

2.11 Bacon Avocado Burger...65

2.12 Spinach Fry Up & Tomato Mushroom..65

2.13 Chocolate Milkshake..66

2.14 Almond Sweet Cherry Chia Pudding...67

2.15 Shakshuka..67

2.16 Anti-Inflammatory Salad..68

2.17 Amaranth Porridge with Pears...69

2.18 Sweet Potato Breakfast Container...69

2.19 Apple Turkey Hash...70

2.20 Oats with Almonds and Blueberries...71

2.21 Chia Energy Bars with Chocolate..71

2.22 Baked Rice Porridge with Maple and Fruit...72

2.23 Banana Chia Pudding..72

2.24 Baked Eggs with Herbs...73

2.25 Banana Bread Pecan Overnight Oats..73

2.26 Cinnamon Granola with Fruits..74

2.27 Yogurt Parfait with Chia Seeds and Raspberries..74

2.28 Avocado Toast with Egg...75

2.29 Winter Morning Breakfast Container...75

2.30 Broccoli and Quinoa Breakfast Patties...76

2.31 Scrambled Tofu Breakfast Tacos..77

2.32 Potato Skillet Breakfast...77

2.33 Peanut Butter and Banana Bread Granola..78

2.34 Chocolate Chip, Strawberry and Oat Waffles..79

2.35 Chickpea Flour Omelet...79

CHAPTER 3: Anti-Inflammatory Lunch Recipes...81

3.1 Buddha Container with Avocado, Wild Rice, Kale, and Orange...81

3.2 Avocado Chickpea Salad Sandwich..82

3.3 Spiced Lentil Soup..83

3.4 Red Lentil Pasta with Tomato..84

3.5 Tuna Mediterranean Salad..84

3.6 Chicken and Greek Salad Wrap..85

3.7 Cauliflower and Chickpea Coconut Curry...86

3.8 Butternut Squash Carrot Soup...87

3.9 Kale Quinoa Shrimp Container...87

3.10 Egg Container and Veggies..88

3.11 Turkey Taco Containers..89

3.12 Bulgur Kale Pesto Salad...90

3.13 Turkish Scrambled Eggs...91

3.14 Swiss Chard and Red Lentil Curried Soup...91

3.15 Orange Cardamom Quinoa with Carrots..92

3.16 Quinoa Turmeric Power Container...93

3.17 Tomato Stew with Chickpea and Kale...93

3.18 Anti-Inflammatory Beef Meatballs..94

3.19 Salmon with Veggies Sheet Pan...94

3.20 Roasted Salmon Garlic and Broccoli...95

3.21 Roasted Sweet Potatoes with Avocado Dip..96

3.22 Chicken with Lemon and Asparagus...96

3.23 Lentil Soup with Lemons..97

3.24 Shrimp Fajitas...98

3.25 Mediterranean One Pan Cod..98

3.26 Garlic Tomato Basil Chicken...99

3.27 Asian Garlic Noodles...100

3.28 Shrimp Garlic Zoodles..101

3.29 Cauliflower Grits and Shrimp..101

3.30 Green Curry..102

CHAPTER 4: Anti-Inflammatory Dinner Recipes...103

4.1 Stir-Fried Snap Pea and Chicken...103

4.2 Turkey Chili with Avocado...104

4.3 Turkey Burgers with Tzatziki Sauce...104

4.4 Fried Rice with Pineapple...105

4.5 Ratatouille...106

4.6 Eggs with Tomatoes and Asparagus...107

4.7 Turmeric, Carrot, and Ginger Soup...107

4.8 Bulgur and Sweet Potato Salad..108

4.9 Salmon Roast with Romaine and Potatoes..109

4.10 Bean Bolognese..110

4.11 Peppers Stuffed with Sweet Potato and Turkey..110

4.12 Turkey Meatballs...111

4.13 Chicken Chili and White Beans..111

4.14 Cauliflower Rice and Salmon Container...112

4.15 Harissa and Chicken Tsideers...113

4.16 Chinese Chicken Salad..114

4.17 Baked Cauliflower Buffalo..114

4.18 Kale and Sweet Potato Tostadas...115

CHAPTER 5: Anti-Inflammatory Snack Recipes..116

5.1 Spicy Tuna Rolls...116

5.2 Turmeric Gummies..117

5.3 Ginger-Cinnamon Mixed Nuts...117

5.4 Ginger Date Almond Bars...118

5.5 Coffee Cacao Protein Bars...*118*

Conclusion...**120**

INTERMITTENT FASTING FOR WOMEN OVER 60

Introduction

The golden decade is a wonderful moment for a woman. They accept themselves thoroughly and attempt to live a happy and peaceful life. Wouldn't it be wonderful if that was the case all of the time? Unfortunately, it isn't, and although women may have a good life beyond 60, several problems can put a stop to their lifestyle. As women age, their body form naturally changes. They typically start to put on weight once they hit the age of 60. Weight loss tends to happen later in life, partially due to fat replacing lean muscle tissues. A good diet can play a major impact in a woman's body transition in their life. Women over the age of 60 may encounter difficulties when attempting to lose weight. Often, the primary factor is a slowed metabolism. A women's metabolism will be faster if they have more lean muscle. Women can influence the aging process rate by altering their ways of life. One of the things to do to slow down the aging process in the body includes Intermittent fasting (IF). Intermittent fasting has attracted increasing attention in recent years due to the variety of health benefits it provides and the fact that it does not limit food choices. Intermittent fasting helps improve metabolism and mental wellbeing and may even help prevent certain cancers. It can also help women over 60 avoid specific nerve, muscle, and joint disorders. It is not a diet but rather a way of life. This diet will help you eat fewer calories on a daily basis and will assist you in going on with your weight loss journey. Certain women practicing IF opt for alternate-day fasting in, which they normally eat on alternate days and consume only 25% of their usual daily calorie intake on the rest of the days. Others prefer their eating patterns according to the hrs of the day.

Intermittent fasting has plenty of other benefits for women in their 60s. Intermittent fasting also helps lower insulin resistance, resulting in a 20-30% reduction in blood sugar and fasting insulin levels, potentially protecting from type 2 diabetes, especially in women over 60. Several studies indicate that IF reduces inflammatory indicators, which are a major contributor to the development of many chronic illnesses. Intermittent fasting also reduces cholesterol, which contributes to heart disease. Apart from physical benefits, IF promotes a healthier mentality. It stimulates brain chemicals that help create new brain cells that combat Alzheimer's disease and promote clarity of thought for women. Intermittent fasting is a perfect way for a woman to start their 60s and feel confident like never before.

Chapter 1: What Happens To A Women's Body After 60

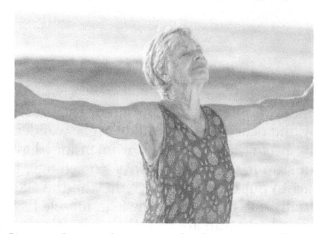

As women age, their bodies undergo changes, which are not always harmful - they are just different. Learning what to expect will assist in accepting these changes and understanding what to do to smooth the transition. While some of these transformations are imperceptible and occur gradually, others tend to happen rapidly. Whatever time they occur; it is important to understand that they are natural.

1.1 Metabolism System of Women over 60

Over the age of 60, one encounters difficulties while attempting to reduce weight. This is a major problem among women. It might be a result of a variety of factors. Often, the core problem is decreased metabolism. Metabolic rate begins to decline in women at the age of 60s after a rapid rise in teens and early twenties before ultimately leveling out in fifties. Over the age of 60, metabolism slows down. Metabolism can get better by gaining more lean muscle. However, as women age, they drop lean muscle mass and frequently are much less active than they once were. As a result, Stubborn body fat that simply would not leave occurs. To get rid of this problem, fasting has been shown to boost metabolism and emotional health and help avoid some malignancies.

A slowed metabolism can be caused by various factors, including

- Consuming excessive fat, which the body attempts to store by lowering the metabolic system.
- Consuming insufficient calories causes a woman's body to slow down since it assumes that the person is starving.
- A lack of physical activity might result in abdominal fat.
- Certain medicines, such as steroids, diabetic medications, and antidepressants, can cause slowed metabolism in women.
- Medical issues such as thyroid that are no longer functioning or the insulin that is no longer usable.

Any of these may be contributing factors to slowed metabolism, which might result in surprising weight gain in the long run.

1.2 HGH Production Level in Women

A crucial factor in reducing the aging process is the human growth hormone (HGH). A women's body in the 60 produces less testosterone, estrogen, and human growth hormone (HGH), which results in muscle loss - and muscle is a critical component of a healthy metabolism. A recent study has proven that HGH has a direct favorable effect on various biological functions. The pituitary gland secretes HGH during sleep and has a role in tissue healing, cell replication, and bone health. However, by the time women reach their sixties, their overall HGH levels will be around half of what they were at twenty. As a result of the decreased HGH production, you will have significantly decreased endurance, more body fat, a longer healing period, and a compromised immune system. Although HGH production declines with age, some beneficial lifestyle modifications might help naturally increase HGH production for women over 60's.

The most prevalent signs of adult growth hormone insufficiency in women over 60's are as follows:

- Metabolic abnormalities in the central region (belly fat)
- Depression
- Decreased Mineral Density of the Bone
- Muscle mass loss
- Anxiety
- Insulin sensitivity is decreased
- Hypercholesterolemia
- Dysfunction of the neuromuscular system
- Decreased strength
- Muscle mass loss

Additionally, genetics may have a role in developing a deficiency. On the other hand, a significant proportion of female hormone deficiency is caused by a pituitary adenoma or its therapy (surgery, radiation, etc.). Over the last several decades, it has been shown that HGH shortage is also caused by women participating in contact sports such as basketball, rugby and boxing, and other activities that can result in traumatic brain damage and head trauma, resulting in adult GHD. According to studies, fasting results in a significant boost in HGH levels of women over 60. One researcher discovered that HGH levels jump by more than 300 percent three days into a fast, grown by a staggering 1,250 percent after a week of fasting. Other studies have discovered comparable results, with HGH levels doubling or tripling after only 2–3 days of fasting. On the other hand, continuous fasting is not sustainable in the long run. Intermittent fasting is an increasingly prevalent dietary strategy that restricts eating to small time intervals.

There are several techniques of intermittent fasting. A frequent technique is to alternate a daily eight-hour eating window with a sixteen-hour fast. Another includes consuming 500–600 calories twice a week. Intermittent fasting can aid in the optimization of HGH levels in two ways. To begin, it can assist in losing body fat, which has a direct effect on HGH production. Secondly, insulin is released while eating, which will keep insulin levels low for most of the day. Insulin surges may disrupt the body's natural growth hormone production. Significant changes in HGH levels occur between fasting and feeding days. 12–16-hour fasts are likely beneficial for HGH production.

1.3 Other Effects of Aging:

Cardiovascular System

As women grow old, their heart and blood arteries grow stiffer, and the heart fills with blood at a slower rate than it did previously. Women over 60's are more likely than younger women to acquire high blood pressure because the stiffer the blood vessels are, the less room there is for blood vessels to expand as blood is pushed through them. A typical older heart is still functional, but it cannot pump as much blood as a younger heart or accelerate as rapidly as a younger heart. As women get older, they might experience changes in their heart and blood arteries. When a woman reaches middle age, for instance, her heart is unable to beat as rapidly as it did when she was younger, even in stressful situations or when she was engaging in strenuous physical activity. The amount of times that the heart beats in a min, often known as the heart rate, doesn't, nevertheless, change drastically as a typical part of the aging process. Because of all of the medical advancements that have occurred in the previous two decades, the number of deaths from heart-related disorders has decreased significantly. As women age, the heart and arteries become stiffer, making it even more crucial to do everything they can to maintain their cardiovascular system as healthy as possible. Physical exercise, such as any form of aerobic activity and a good diet, are excellent strategies.

Immune System

By reaching the decade, the immune system begins to function less effectively. It might result in the following issues:

- The chance of becoming sick increases due to the immune system's tendency to respond more slowly to stimuli.
- There is a possibility that vaccines such as the flu and pneumonia jabs will no longer be effective or last as long as they once did.
- With aging, a women's body recovers more slowly since they have fewer immune cells to fight off infection.
- The capacity of the body to identify and fix flaws in cells diminishes while growing older and increasing the chance of acquiring cancer.
- Women can develop an autoimmune illness, a condition in which the immune system targets and kills healthy bodily tissue by mistake.

It is essential to take good care to ensure that the immune system is as healthy as possible. Receiving the vaccinations the doctor recommends, such as those for the flu (get a high-dose flu vaccine if 60 or older), pneumococcal disease, pneumonia, and shingles. Eating a proper diet, exercising regularly, abstaining from smoking, and limiting your alcohol use will help maintain the immune system in good shape.

Declining Bone Mass

Aging is caused by a variety of functional changes that result in a significant loss in all human capacities. With aging, a range of anatomical and functional changes occur. Declining bone mass is a common concern among women over the age of 60. A woman's bones begin to lose protein matrix tissue after she has gone through menopause, resulting in increased deformation of the bones. Bone mass reaches its maximum at the age of 35 and then begins to decline as levels of estrogen decline. Women often break bones in accidents when they are in their 60s, resulting in a huge bruise, while this would have hardly affected them in their 30s.

Chapter 2: What Is Intermittent Fasting?

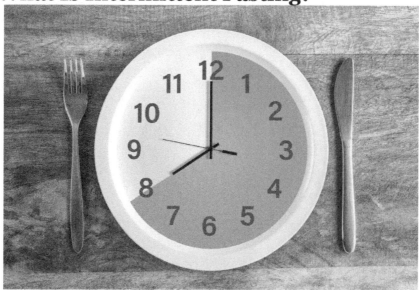

Intermittent fasting has become a popular weight-loss approach; it is not a new phenomenon. Apart from religious and spiritual motives, fasting has been practiced by numerous civilizations throughout history to improve physical and mental health. The ancient Greek athletes, for example, would fast to prepare themselves for competition in the Olympic games. But what precisely is intermittent fasting, and how does it differ from regular fasting? And more importantly, can restricting food consumption to particular intervals of the day or certain days of a week truly help lose weight? Following is the answer to these questions. Intermittent fasting (IF) is a diet that sticks to a schedule that alternates between eating times and intervals of not eating. It is an eating approach that does not place restrictions on what one eats but on when one consumes it. Intermittent fasting for weight reduction has been shown to enhance metabolic health and reduce insulin levels in women, allowing the body to burn more calories throughout the day.

Many different techniques for intermittent fasting exist; however, all of them revolve around alternating times of eating with periods of fasting. Choosing to eat at specific times of the day or on particular days of the week is permissible as long as the routine is consistent. Unlike other diets, which instruct on what to eat, intermittent fasting instructs when to eat by introducing frequent short-term fasts into the routine. A low-calorie diet may help lose weight while also lowering the chances of developing diabetes and heart disease. Unlike other diets, intermittent fasting does not keep track of the calories or macronutrient consumption. There are no restrictions on which foods must be consumed or avoided, making it more like a lifestyle than a diet. Many individuals utilize intermittent fasting to lose weight because it is an easy, practical, and successful strategy to consume less and shed body fat while maintaining energy levels. It also aids in the prevention of heart diseases and diabetes, the preservation of muscular mass, and the improvement of psychological well-being. Furthermore, it has fewer meals to plan, prepare, and cook. This eating pattern might help save time in the kitchen.

2.1 Benefits of Intermittent Fasting for Women over 60's

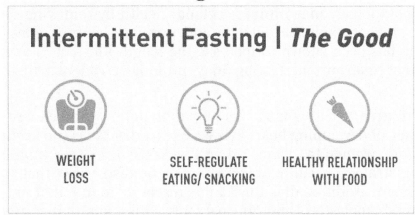

The benefits of intermittent fasting are not just derived from eating less (although this may occur when limiting the window of food availability) but also from metabolic changes that occur when spending long periods without eating. The word autophagy is used to describe the fundamental adaption that occurs during a fast. Autophagy is the body's self-cleansing function, which activates when nutrients are insufficiently accessible to the cells. It is necessary to clear away damaged or old cells to create a place for better cells to maintain cellular and metabolic health. Autophagy has been linked to the avoidance of chronic illness and increased lifespan. Given that autophagy activity usually declines with age, fasting may be a natural strategy to boost it. Autophagy is one of the benefits of intermittent fasting, but there are other more intriguing study discoveries, such as the following:

Weight Loss: Large number of research has shown the effectiveness of intermittent fasting for weight reduction in women over 60's. Some study shows that women who follow intermittent fasting routines lose the same amount of weight as those who decrease calories without experiencing feelings of deprivation. In terms of helping women over 60 lose weight and eliminate extra body fat, intermittent fasting is a beneficial lifestyle decision. According to various research papers, adopting an intermittent fasting diet resulted in an average weight reduction of 15 pounds on average. Another thorough assessment of the studies on intermittent fasting discovered that it might decrease the bodyweight of overweight women by up to 8% in as little as three weeks when done consistently.

Increased Fat Burning in Women over 60's: While reducing carbohydrate consumption, the body begins to use other energy sources as a substitute. After using up all carbohydrate reserves, it might turn to fat for fuel. According to some studies, fasting boosts fat burning by activating the metabolic switch, which allows fat to be used as fuel. Consuming food within a certain time frame causes the body to burn more calories during the rest of its working day. Because the longer without eating, the slower the metabolism gets. However, by restricting the meal consumption to an 8-hour timeframe, a woman's body will step up to the plate and burn more calories throughout the day and night.

The state of one's mind: Fasting may help to improve cognitive performance, which is particularly important as women reach their 60s. It may also slow down neurodegeneration, which is the steady deterioration of brain cells over time, but this has only been shown in preclinical studies. Several modifiable factors influence cognitive health and the risk of cognitive decline and Alzheimer's disease. These factors include blood glucose and insulin levels and other metabolic and lipid profiles. Intermittent fasting has been proven to improve several of these factors, which may also positively affect cognition.

Recent experiments have also shown that fasting on an intermittent basis may be beneficial to the neurologic health of women in their 60s.

Longevity: Since autophagy may promote cellular health by removing old, damaged cells, it may be able to prevent oxidative damage and promote healthy aging in the long run. Intermittent fasting has been shown to increase the length lifespan in women. Researchers have discovered that intermittent fasting may prolong a rodent's lifetime by 33-88 in women.

Cardiovascular health: Fasting may also help to maintain good cholesterol levels, which may lower the chance of developing heart disease. Heart disease is the leading cause of death globally, killing more women than any other illness. Within two months of starting an intermittent fasting strategy, a study of women over 60 discovered that it decreased blood pressure by 6 percent. Additionally, this same research found that intermittent fasting reduced participants' cholesterol by 25 percent while simultaneously lowering their triglycerides by an incredible 32 percent

Insulin resistance and high blood sugar levels: Another benefit is that fasting may be as effective as a calorie-restricted diet for promoting weight loss, insulin production, and insulin resistance reduction, according to research. By decreasing insulin levels and drastically reducing insulin resistance, intermittent fasting may help women reduce their chance of acquiring diabetes in the first place. In a study of 100 women over 60's, intermittent fasting for only six months lowered insulin levels by 29 percent and insulin resistance by 19 percent, respectively. Studies conducted on healthy individuals have established the magic of intermittent fasting to reduce insulin levels by 21-31 percent and blood sugar levels by 3-6 percent in women with pre-diabetes in about 8-12 weeks has been established in studies conducted on healthy individuals.

Immunity: Through the process of autophagy, fasting may have a beneficial effect on the creation of healthy white blood cells. Irregular fasting is an excellent immune system regulator because it regulates the quantity of cytokine production that is released into the bloodstream. The cytokines interleukin-6 and tumor necrosis factor-alpha, two of the most important in the body's inflammatory response, work together. According to research, fasting has been demonstrated to inhibit the release of these inflammatory mediators. The immune system modulation that intermittent fasting offers may also be beneficial for women who suffer from moderate to severe allergies.

Inflammation: Inflammation is a medical term that refers to the body's inflammation. Several studies have shown that fasting positively affects inflammation and oxidative stress indicators. Intermittent fasting may be more effective than other diets when it comes to decreasing inflammation and improving disorders that are related to inflammation, such as:

- Alzheimer's disease is a kind of dementia.
- Arthritis
- Asthma
- Multiple sclerosis is a disease that affects the nervous system.
- Stroke

Maintain lean muscular tone: Fasting has been shown to assist in maintaining lean muscular tone. Compared to calorie-restricted diets, studies have demonstrated that intermittent fasting is more successful in retaining lean muscle mass than other diets for women over 60's.

Having a healthy amount of lean muscle tone makes the body more fit and appealing and allows it to burn much more calories - even when the body is fully at rest. This is a major benefit of fasting which can help a lot of women over 60 gain confidence.

Psychological and emotional well-being: Another benefit of intermittent fasting is one's psychological and emotional well-being. According to the findings of recent research, merely 8 weeks of intermittent fasting may significantly reduce depression and binge eating behaviors in women in their 60s while simultaneously improving levels of self-esteem. Many women feel happier after fasting, resulting into a better life.

2.2 The Truth about Intermittent Fasting

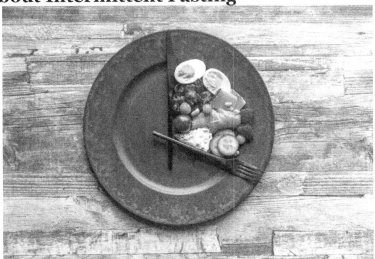

Intermittent fasting is a fantastic strategy to lose weight, and to a certain degree, it may also help enhance metabolic activity. However, according to the data of many researchers, it is not a more effective or faster method of reducing weight when compared to daily calorie restriction but definitely a healthier one. It is necessary to make lifestyle modifications to practice intermittent fasting, and time-restricted fasting is the most practicable strategy for working professionals. Additionally, intermittent fasting has several health advantages, which may be enhanced even further if being mindful of the food intake throughout the non-fasting time. Eat high-calorie junk food during the non-fasting window, and the benefits of intermittent fasting may be diminished due to the additional calories consumed. Maintaining a 16-hour fast and consuming high-calorie items such as fries, chips, cakes, and other baked goods may undermine all of the work to maintain a fast. To want to transition to intermittent fasting, make sure to have a well-balanced and healthy meal during the periods when you are not fasting. For the first few days, it may be difficult to stick to an intermittent fasting schedule since the body is not used to being hungry for such a long time. But if being persistive towards it, the body will develop the habit of missing breakfast for a few of days. Sipping on a cup of black coffee or green tea in the morning will satisfy hunger if particularly hungry. Although these beverages do not promote the production of much insulin, these drinks may help prolong the fasting state while also reducing hunger symptoms.

The truth is that intermittent fasting is not really a solution, but it may benefit certain people who want to achieve their health objectives while maintaining their eating habits. It may thus be an advantageous lifestyle if one does not have any concerns with cravings, migraines, or low sugar levels while on this diet plan. For a woman experiencing any of these symptoms, it is apparent that this is not a healthy solution. Several different approaches to achieving the health objectives do not need adhering to a diet, but it's an intriguing and promising idea to try intermittent fasting.

Dietary trend may be on their way out as people turn their attention to nutrition rather than calories counted to lose weight. Alternatively, it might represent a significant lifestyle constraint, especially if the body of data is still being debated, and it may also have its own set of potentially harmful side effects. As an emerging idea, intermittent fasting requires a longer period of observation and more human trials before it can be recommended. Please be advised that fasting is not suggested for some groups of individuals, those with a history of eating problems and people with type 1 diabetes. Those considering trying the intermittent fasting diet should speak with their primary care physician and, if possible, with a qualified dietitian before proceedings

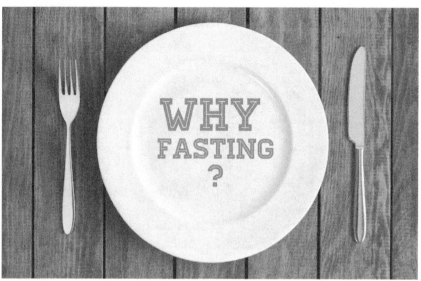

2.3 Why start Intermittent Fasting After the '60s

Many women start practicing intermittent fasting for a variety of different purposes. It might be for several reasons, including weight reduction, improved sleep at night, or increased vitality. One of the most compelling reasons for women over 60 to pursue intermittent fasting is the desire for improved energy. Many women endure a small weight increase and a decrease in the quality of their sleep in their 60s. Both have the potential to make the body feel tired and unproductive. However, by altering the timing and composition of meals, women can retrain the body to function more efficiently. While fasting to lose weight, intermittent fasting may enable consuming the things that a woman desires when craving them the most — in the middle of the night. In other words, feeling starved when everyone else is nibbling in front of the television while watching their favorite shows will be over.

2.4 How is Intermittent Fasting Riskier for Women over 60?

While beginning any form of fast, as with any other substantial change in eating habits, one should first consult with a healthcare practitioner. Even mild fasting may be dangerous, particularly for women who have a history of eating disorders or disordered eating patterns.

- Having diabetes or hypoglycemia may be dangerous, particularly if using drugs that reduce blood sugar.
- Women who are having difficulty gaining enough weight or who are dealing with vitamin deficits.

- A history of electrolyte abnormalities, particularly after fasting for extended periods.

It's not that some women cannot fast if they fall into any of these categories, but it is much more crucial to seek professional counsel to determine whether or not it is safe for them to do so. No words can express how important it is to consult with a trained health practitioner before commencing if diagnosed with a history of disordered eating or an eating disorder. It is possible that the anticipated danger will not occur. Stress has a significant influence on women's hormones, which accounts for a big portion of the reasons why fasting might be different for them. Intermittent fasting is generally considered to be safe for the majority of individuals. However, investigations have shown that intermittent fasting has certain mild bad impacts. Furthermore, it is not the best option for everyone. The following are the risks of Intermittent Fasting for women in their 60s.

Migraines and dizziness: Intermittent fasting is associated with several unpleasant side effects, including headaches. They are most often experienced during the first several days of a diet program. A study published in 2022 looked at numerous studies, including women over 60 who were on intermittent fasting regimens. Some individuals in the four trials that recorded negative impacts felt slight headaches. Contrary to popular belief, however, studies have discovered that "fasting headaches" are frequently situated in the brain's frontal area, with the severity of the pain normally being mild to moderate. Furthermore, those who suffer from headaches regularly are more prone than those who do not to suffer from headaches when fasting. Researchers have hypothesized that low caffeine withdrawal and low blood sugar may play a role in headaches in women over 60 s when intermittent fasting.

Exhaustion and a lack of energy: According to studies, some women who follow different techniques of intermittent fasting report exhaustion and a lack of energy on certain occasions. If you suffer from severe adrenal exhaustion, intermittent fasting may make you feel weak. Because your body doesn't have enough adrenaline to control your blood sugar, intermittent fasting might produce low blood sugar (hypoglycemia). Feeling fatigued and weak due to low blood sugar caused by intermittent fasting is common in women. In addition, intermittent fasting may induce sleep difficulties in certain women, resulting in fatigue throughout the day for those who follow it. However, several studies have shown that intermittent fasting might actually help to lessen tiredness, particularly when the body gets used to regular fasting intervals.

Hunger pangs: It may come as no surprise that hunger is one of the most prominent negative outcomes associated with intermittent fasting for women over 60's, as it is with any other kind of diet. Women may feel an increased appetite when restricting their calorie intake or going for long durations without consuming calories. Some women in a research were allocated to an intermittent energy restriction group. They ate 440 or 650 calories on two nonconsecutive days per week for a year, depending on their weight. Participants in these groups reported greater hunger levels than those who followed a low-calorie diet that included continual calorie restriction. Scientists believe that hunger is a symptom that individuals feel during the first few days of starting a fasting program. Another research from 2020 looked at 15 women over 60's who took part in fasting programs that lasted between 4 and 21 days. When they started the regimens, they tended to have severe hunger sensations during the first several days. As a result, sensations such as hunger may subside as the body gets used to frequent fasting intervals.

Inability to control one's temper and other mood swings: Women over 60 who practice intermittent fasting may develop irritation and other mood problems due to their efforts. When the blood sugar is low, women may get irritable. It is possible to have low blood sugar, or hypoglycemia, during times of calorie restriction or during periods of fasting.

This might result in irritation, anxiety, and difficulty concentrating on tasks. Research published in 2020 on 52 women over 60 discovered that participants were substantially more irritable after an 18-hour fasting phase than they were during a no fasting time. Interestingly, the researchers discovered that, although the women were more irritable after the fasting period, they also reported a greater feeling of accomplishment, pride, and self-control at the side of the fasting period than they did at the beginning of the fasting period.

Bad Breath

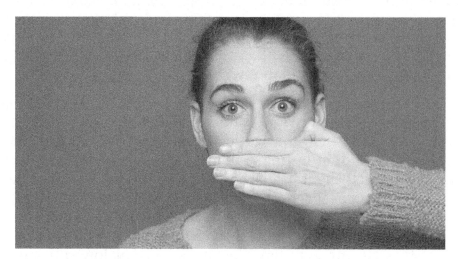

In certain women, bad breath may be a nasty side effect of intermittent fasting, which can be particularly uncomfortable. This is caused by a loss of salivary flow and an increase in the amount of acetone in the breath. Fasting helps your body to burn fat as fuel, which is beneficial. Acetone is a by-product of fat metabolism, and as a result, it accumulates in the blood and exhaled breath while fasting. Dehydration is also a side effect of intermittent fasting and may also produce dry mouth, exacerbating foul breath.

Digestive problems: Symptoms of intermittent fasting include diarrhea, nausea, bloating and constipation. While fasting, the decrease in food consumption associated with certain intermittent fasting regimens may severely impact digestion, resulting in constipation and other adverse effects. Furthermore, dietary modifications connected with intermittent fasting routines may result in bloating and diarrhea. Constipation might worsen due to dehydration, which is another typical adverse effect of intermittent fasting. As a result, it is critical to maintaining enough hydration when engaging in intermittent fasting. Constipation may be prevented by eating meals that are high in nutrients and fiber.

Disturbed Sleep

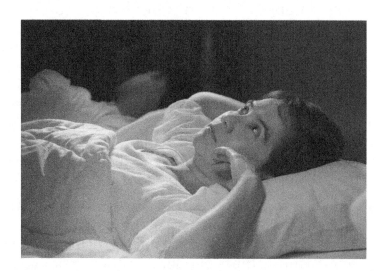

While intermittent fasting tend to increase sleep quality, depending on how meals are timed, it may also cause sleep problems. Women' s sleep might be disrupted when they eat at odd hrs. This is particularly true if individuals eat late at night, since this may cause the body's temperature to rise, which is the polar opposite of what happens when sleeping. Heavy meals eaten too soon at night may upset the stomach and make it difficult to fall asleep, resulting in poor sleep quality and a lack of energy when one wakes up. Moreover, Sleep disruptions, such as the inability to fall asleep or remain asleep, are among the most prevalent negative effects associated with intermittent fasting, such as insomnia for women over 60. As the body excretes huge quantities of salt and water via the urine during the first few days of an intermittent fasting diet, fatigue may be more typical during those first few days. Dehydration and low sodium levels might occur as a result. Other research, on the other hand, has shown that intermittent fasting has no impact on sleep in women over 60's.

Dehydration: During the first few days of fasting, the body excretes enormous volumes of water and salt via the urine, which is a sign of dehydration. Natural diuresis, also known as natriuretic of fasting, is the term used to describe this process. If this occurs and does not replenish the fluids and electrolytes lost through urine, the person may become dehydrated. In addition, women who practice intermittent fasting may forget to drink or may not drink enough water during their fasting periods. This is particularly likely to occur at the start of an intermittent fasting routine. To get through a lengthy fast, many individuals depside on caffeine in coffee (or flavored coffee). While this isn't always a problem, the fact remains that coffee is a diuretic. In other words, it has the potential to cause dehydration. That's why drink plenty of water throughout the day and keep an eye on the urine color to ensure that the body is well hydrated. A light lemonade hue is an ideal choice for this. If your urine is dark in color, it may indicate that you are dehydrated.

Poor Nutrition: Intermittent fasting, if not done appropriately, may result in nutritional deficiency. It is possible to become malnourished if a woman fasts for an extended length of time and do not refill their body with sufficient nutrients. Women who participate in different forms of intermittent fasting programs can often satisfy their calorie and nutritional requirements. However, if someone doesn't properly plan and implement the fasting program over a long time, or if they purposely limit calories to an excessive degree, they may suffer from malnutrition and other health problems. It is important to have a well-balanced, healthy diet when engaging in intermittent fasting. Make certain not to restrict calorie intake excessively. A healthcare practitioner with extensive knowledge in intermittent fasting can assist at the start of intermittent fasting in developing a safe strategy that offers a suitable number of calories and the proper quantities of nutrients for your specific nutritional needs. However, many of these symptoms can be reduced by making modest modifications, such as reducing the length of time to fast. Having said that, some individuals just do not feel good when fasting, and which is perfectly acceptable.

The disadvantages outweigh the advantages.

If you've come this far and decide to fast, it's a good idea to think about how you can do it securely. Here are some steps you can take to get started.

Begin with little steps. If you've never fasted before, you shouldn't go into an extensive fast without some preparation. Begin by simply extending the time between supper and breakfast by a few mins more than customary. Even ten hrs is wonderful if you're used to grazing throughout the evening. Because digestion and insulin function generally slow down as the day progresses, it may be good to start eating supper one hour earlier than you are used to each evening.

Make sure you drink plenty of water. While fasting may imply that you don't consume any calories, calorie-free fluids such as water and herbal tea are advised. Drinking plenty of water can alleviate headaches and hunger pangs in some people. Furthermore, since we satisfy a portion of our overall fluid requirements via water-containing meals, you may need to drink more to make up for lost fluids depending on how long your fast lasts.

Make a plan ahead of time. Make sure you have delicious, healthful things ready to eat when you decide to break your fast. Choose a lunch that is high in healthy fats, protein, and complex carbohydrates for optimum blood sugar balance, and use that meal to set the tone for the remainder of the day. As a source of inspiration, you may consult our free hormone balancing recipe guide.

Keep physical activity to a bare minimum. The length of your fast may dictate how much of an increase in intensity you should do throughout your workout session. Shorter fasts may not necessarily impair your capacity to exercise, but lengthier fasts may need the use of walking or easy yoga as a substitute for vigorous activity.

Pay attention to your body. You're not feeling well when you're fasting? Don't try to push it. If you aren't feeling well, there is simply no need for you to continue your fasting regimen. You are the most knowledgeable about your own body. Don't try to push it; repeat after me.

Chapter 3: Types Of Intermittent Fasting

There are numerous intermittent fasting strategies, ranging in the fasting period: from a twelve-hour overnight fast to a whole-day fast. Methods with a shorter fasting time are well-suited for newbies. Longer fasting times give additional rewards and are suggested for experienced fasters. The first step is to figure out how to make intermittent fasting work for oneself, especially when it comes to things like going out with friend or exercising, so that you don't miss out on important things. Following are different types of intermittent fasting that you can follow.

3.1 A weekly 24-hour Fast

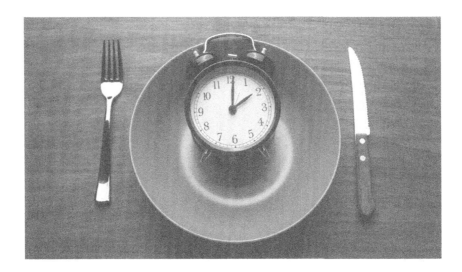

This intermittent fasting pattern, also known as the Eat-Stop-Eat diet, entails going without meals for periods of up to 24 hrs at a time. Many individuals fast from one meal to the next, such as from breakfast to breakfast or lunch to lunch. On days when one is not fasting, one may eat according to a normal schedule. A person's overall calorie intake is reduced due to eating in this way, but the particular items that the individual eats are not restricted. A 24-hour fast may be very difficult because of the weariness, headaches, and irritation that may accompany it. But people get used to this new dietary pattern over time, and they begin to enjoy the advantages as a result. Weekly 24-hour fasting is one of the most popular methods of adopting intermittent fasting into one's lifestyle. It entails limiting food and drink consumption for a whole day (24 hrs) once every week but still consuming all of the nutrients the body requires on all the other days of the week. When one fasts for 24 hrs, they can reflect on themselves and practice self-discipline without experiencing any negative consequences of long periods of fasting, such as hunger or dehydration, that can occur with long periods of absence from food and liquid consumption. It is significant to mention that those who are fasting for 24 hrs may continue to consume water, tea, and other calorie-free beverages throughout their fasting time. It is a crucial component of this diet plan. This may seem to be a difficult task. However, breaking it down into smaller steps is pretty manageable. In the evening before the fasting day, one can eat supper and retire for the night. As soon as the supper is complete, the 24-hour fast period will officially start. The fast for the week is fulfilled the next day when one skips breakfast and lunch and then has a wonderful nutritious supper to round off the day.

After a non-fasting day, one must return to their usual eating habits and resume their normal meal times.

Eating in this manner decreases a person's overall calorie consumption without restricting the kind of meals that the individual eats.

Pros: The benefits of a 24-hour fast include the fact that it is straightforward to follow and its effectiveness in aiding with weight reduction. It puts courage and mental fortitude to the test.

Cons: A 24-hour fast may be draining and exhausting, and it can also produce weariness and headaches. Some individuals discover that their body's response to their new dietary patterns becomes less dramatic over time as they grow used to their new eating habits. Beginning with little steps is the greatest way to succeed: attempt skipping one meal every day till having the motivation to spending a complete day without consuming anything at all. This following kind might be appropriate if one desire's to live a better lifestyle but isn't sure where to begin with.

3.2 12 hrs a day Fast

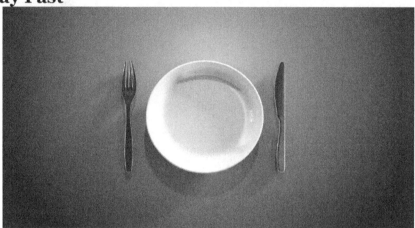

In this type followers typically fast for half of the day and then feast for the rest of the 12-hour period of the day. In addition, the hrs are flexible. From 8.30 am to 8:30 p.m., 10 am to 10:00 pm, and so on, one may eat at any time. The individual must decide to keep the period that has fast. This category of intermittent fasting is ideal for those who are just getting started. The fasting gap is somewhat shorter than usual. The majority of fasting takes place after the night has gone. It is possible to devour it all at the same moment. For example, one might fast between 6:00 p.m. and 6:00 a.m. or between 6:00 pm and 6:00 a.m. They would have to eat their meal by 6 p.m. and then wait for the next day to start. Also, considering that one sleeps 7 to 9 hrs out of those twelve hrs, this type is pretty straightforward to complete. The person who is fasting will likely be sleeping at a time when she may relax. The quickest and most convenient approach to complete the fast is to sleep throughout the timeframe. Finally, the 12-Hour Fast is advised as an excellent starting point for those who are new to intermittent fasting.

Pros: Since it has a smaller period, this style of fasting is simpler to adhere to than others. It may also be beneficial for people who are currently experiencing difficulty sleeping at night and looking for a different solution to enhance their sleep quality.

Cons: Because the fasting period is shorter (just 12 hrs), some individuals may not see the same weight-loss advantages as others who engage in lengthier fasting regimens. This kind of intermittent fasting may also cause weariness, particularly if you are exercising when you are not permitted to eat anything.

3.3 Fasting for 16 hrs

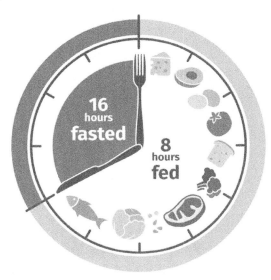

Known as the "birthplace of intermittent fasting," Martin Berkhan developed Leangains in the year 2000. As well as "the Khan, godfather, or high priest of intermittent fasting," Martin is also known as "the Khan." Leangains recommends that one should consume all of the daily calories in 8 hrs and fast for the rest of the 16 hrs of the day. It is the case designed primarily for fitness and strength training and those wishing to achieve the best potential body composition and strength. Compared to other intermittent fasting-based diets, a greater focus is placed on good nutrition before and after workouts. This involves eating higher-protein foods and consuming more calories on training days while consuming fewer calories on rest days, among other things. The 16:8 fasting method is one of the most popular kinds of intermittent fasting since it is simple to implement into one's everyday routine. In this diet one confines their eating to an eight-hour window with two to three meals and then fast for 16 hrs. Example: Eat till 7 pm after supper, then delay breakfast till 11 am the next day, then eat for 8 hrs, and the process begins all over again. In this diet we may adjust the time that suits our needs. One may want to eat sooner or later in the day, depending on the schedule. This sort of fasting is quite simple and is highly recommended for most women in their 60s. The fast is normally completed by 7 p.m. with supper, and the following day, there is no breakfast eaten by the participants. There will be no food served till noon. This intermittent fasting may also be beneficial for those who have previously attempted the 12 Hour Fast and were disappointed by the outcomes. According to studies, restricting the feeding period to 8 hrs kept them from developing obesity and inflammation and liver disease in the same proportion as when they ate the same amount of calories as before. Diets such as the Leangains diet might be effective.

Pros: Intermittent fasting of this sort is an excellent alternative for people who have previously tried the 12 Hour Fast but have not seen significant weight reduction results. It may also aid in muscle repair and the management of low blood glucose after exercises, including a few of the advantages.

Cons: This kind of fast is not recommended since it only lasts for a maximum of 16 hrs first before women can eat again. Some individuals may be able to stick to this diet more successfully than others because they do not eat numerous meals throughout the day, which causes them to feel unproductive or exhausted.

3.4 The Warrior Diet

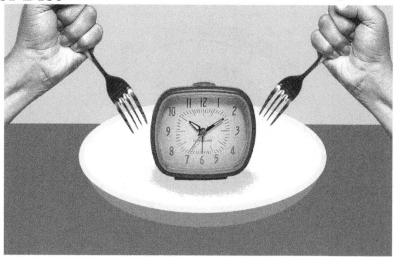

This diet is a twenty-hour fasting phase during which one consumes just a few portion sizes per day before having a huge meal before going to bed. This is a fairly intensive kind of fasting since one is not permitted to consume food or any meals during the day till supper. The body will fast for twenty hrs every day in order to practice the warrior diet, excluding one four-hour eating period where one will eat only healthy foods. This kind of fasting may help with mental clarity, weight loss, stress reduction, and the formation of muscle mass. On the other side, this plan may be too tough for some people to stick to since it requires just a few meals per day and little food on such days. According to its founder, Ori Hofmekler, The Warrior Diet may not be ideal for beginners. The warriors fast for over twenty hrs a day and eat just one heavy meal at night. On the other side, fasting allows only a small number of whole foods, fruits, meats, and vegetables. This diet has been based on common ideas with the Paleo diet. Instead of processed items, it encourages individuals to eat real meals, including meat, chicken, fish, vegetables, and whole grains.

Pros: The fact that a warrior diet is advantageous to overall health in a multitude of ways is one of its many advantages. One of the most sought-after benefits of the warrior diet is its potential to lower risk factors associated with diabetes and high blood pressure. When compared to not fasting at all, this type of intermittent fasting benefits in achieving and maintaining a healthy physique by reducing the chance of binge eating.
Cons: This diet may be tough to continue due to the restricted selection of meals accessible. Consequently, women have a limited eating period, and the diet may be low in some nutrients, such as fiber, as a result of this limitation. The second downside of this lifestyle is that it may be hard to maintain a warrior mindset for long periods, especially when hunger pains appear.

3.5 Alternate Day Fasting

Alternate day fasting is a kind of intermittent fasting taken to the extreme. As the name implies, fasting every other day is part of this regimen. Food is confined to a single 500-calorie meal or complete fasting on fasting days, depending on the situation (without calories). On alternate days, one may eat as they usually would. Alternate day fasting is a difficult type of fasting that is unlikely to be sustained in the long run. Alternate day fasting is a practice in which individuals abstain from eating solid meals on alternate days.

It is important to note that alternate-day fasting is a very severe type of intermittent fasting, and it may not be appropriate for women who have never fasted before or for those who have certain medical concerns. Beginners experiencing medical troubles may wish to avoid using this fasting technique. Additionally, it may be difficult to maintain a consistent fasting approach for an extended period. Some studies, however, have indicated that alternate-day fasting may result in significant weight reduction, improved digestive and immunological health, and improved metabolic health. One research estimated that 32 individuals dropped an average of about 10 pounds over 12 weeks. Over the study's 12 weeks, 32 individuals dropped a total of 5.3 kg. According to reliable sources, it was also proven to be beneficial for reducing weight and improving heart health in healthy and overweight women. For some individuals, an alternative diet is consuming foods that are not solid. **Pros:** This diet may be useful for weight reduction and improving health indicators such as blood pressure and cholesterol levels.

Cons: Even if one is a rookie or has medical concerns that would make this harmful, it is incredibly tough to go through this form of fasting. It may also take up to 12 weeks before one see any noticeable improvements.

3.6 5:2 Method

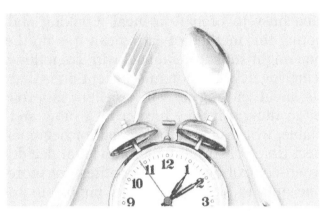

Michael Mosley is recognized for popularizing the 5:2 intermittent fasting method, often referred to as The Fast Diet. This strategy involves restricting calorie intake to 25% of daily needs on 2 days each week while eating properly on the rest of the days. Five days of the week are defined as "normal dining days," as the term indicates. The last two days have calorie limits of 450 to 560 per day. Most people split the two fasting days to avoid the hungry specific symptoms with a two-day fast. During the 2 days of fasting, women intake approximately 400 calories each day. Women usually adhere to this diet by spacing out regular fasting days all week. As a result, individuals may fast on Tuesdays and Friday while eating normally the rest of the week. To ensure proper digestion, at least one free day should be included between fasting days. This diet, sometimes called also as Fast Diet, has gotten very little research attention. The study included 110 women over the age of 60 and found that caloric intake restriction once a week and constant calorie counting both resulted in similar weight loss. Among the most apparent benefits was that blood sugar levels decreased considerably, allowing patients to lose weight and improve.

Pros: This meal plan is easily understandable and has been demonstrated to help people lose weight while also lowering their insulin levels.

Cons: Sticking to this kind of fasting may be more challenging since it may experience hunger and be unable to find food throughout the fast.

3.7 Meal Skipping

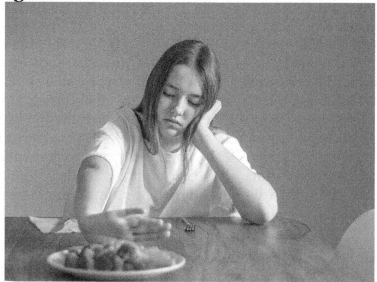

This diet is ideal for individuals who do not want to feel confined or who get disappointed if they do not satisfy the requirements of a certain diet plan. In it just allow oneself to miss meals if not hungry or too busy to prepare a meal. Cooking and eating take up a great amount of time, and adopting this method of eating can free up the time to devote to other activities—for example, one might substitute a meal with something they like doing, such as going on a walk or practicing yoga. A common misconception is that we must eat three meals a day, and spontaneous meal cutting is an excellent approach to deconstruct this assumption. One will not go hungry if they miss a meal now and then! This intermittent fasting technique is adaptable, which may be beneficial for beginners. To maintain a certain degree of hunger or to meet time constraints, the individual decides which meals to forego. Individuals who exercise self-control over their appetites are more likely to be effective at meal switching. When one opts to skip meals, it is important to remember to consume nutritious items while doing so, such as fresh vegetables, to keep the energy levels up.

The simplest approach to describe meal skipping is to say that to eat when hungry and skip meals when are not hungry, as explained above.

Pros: One advantage of missing meals is that it makes it simpler to develop a food plan for the next day. The physical stress on a person's body is reduced since they don't feel as if they have to "do" anything to eat healthfully, and the variety of food selections is almost limitless.

Cons: Cons include individuals reporting feeling hungry or limiting themselves to specific meals during mealtime windows - which might lead to them reverting to their previous eating patterns and routines (eating unhealthy foods). Over time, this form of intermittent fasting does not stimulate weight reduction in the same way that other weight-loss strategies do.

Chapter 4: How to Start Intermittent Fasting?

4.1 Set Your Smart Goals

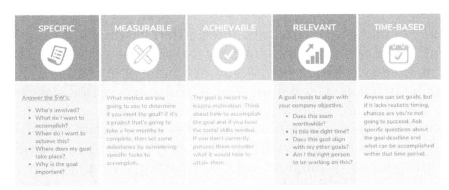

When beginning a new healthy habit, it's vital to consider what obstacles one could encounter. This is an important stage in creating SMART goals, which health coaches use to help clients create realistic, long-term objectives. People have a few frequent issues or questions when it comes to intermittent fasting:

- When I'm not fasting, what do I eat?
- What should I do if I'm feeling queasy or dizzy?
- Is it safe to fast for short periods?
- Should I do an intermittent fast for a certain amount of time?

Understand why you're doing it and assess your current diet

Consider what you want to achieve by incorporating intermittent fasting into your lifestyle:

- Improved dietary habits
- keep track of your blood sugar
- Loss of body weight
- Establish deliberate eating habits, such as eating more thoughtfully.

Whatever your motivation for beginning, examine your present diet and ask yourself what about it is keeping you from achieving the objective you envisioned before. Simple modifications, such as eating a healthy breakfast or learning to calculate macros to better understand portion management, maybe a better first step than plunging right into a fasting habit. You want to discover an eating pattern that works for you rather than dieting and concentrate on developing healthy habits that make you feel your best.

Pick a Time Frame That Matches Your Lifestyle: If you've discussed fasting with your primary care physician and Registered Dietitian and determined that it's a suitable fit for you, be as detailed as possible regarding the kind of fasting and period. As you've read, there are many different sorts of fasting, so sit down and think about your week. Think about your job schedule, sleep pattern, and lifestyle when deciding on a fasting plan.

Begin Small: Start modestly if you're new to occasionally fasting. Choose one day every week to experiment with the style you think would work best for you. For many individuals, short-term fasting is a more sustainable option.

Start with an overnight fast of 8-12 hrs, which is easy to fit into your schedule, then work your way up to lengthier fasting days. If you're going to fast for a long time, choose a day of the week or a period when you won't need to be especially active or concentrated.

Maintain Hydration: Even if you're fasting, you should drink enough no caloric fluids, particularly water, to keep hydrated. Sugar-free herbal teas and sparkly waters may also be included. Half your body weight in oz. is the recommended quantity of water to drink every day. If you weigh 160 pounds, you should drink at least 80 oz. of water every day.

Establish a Meal Preparation Routine: Intermittent fasting, if not done effectively, may lead to weight gain. When you're fasting, you may feel starving, increasing the likelihood that you will engage in excessive eating whilst you are not fasting. Consuming more calories compared to your body burns is going to, over a prolonged period, lead to an increase in body fat, and this is true regardless of whether you fast for twelve to sixteen hrs every day. To put it another way, if you have difficulties controlling your appetite and go fully wild during your non-fasting times, you may gain weight. Plan your meals ahead of time to ensure you have nutrient-dense options throughout your non-fasting hrs and keep below your daily calorie restriction. You should think about what sort of meal plan you love throughout your non-fasting times since intermittent fasting does not substitute good eating. Do you want more plant-based, vegetarian, vegan, or vegetarian meals? Do you want to go keto? Or do you like to strike a balance with a flexitarian diet? Whatever you choose, have a plan for what you'll eat throughout the non-fasting time.

Make a point of eating well-balanced meals: When intermittent fasting, the quality of your meal is critical and controlling your blood sugar might be the key to success. Plan your meals ahead of time to ensure you eat nutrient-dense foods throughout your non-fasting hrs. Ensure you're getting all of the nutrients you need to keep your body going while you're fasting! Consuming meals that are balanced with nutritious whole foods, proteins, and fats regularly throughout your non-fasting phase to keep you full and content while avoiding processed sweets and carbs. You may also attempt intuitive eating, which shifts your attention away from calories and willpower and toward understanding what your body needs to flourish, independent of the time of day or when your next allowed eating window is. To set yourself up for success, remember to integrate fundamental nutrition concepts such as calorie management and a balanced diet, whatever your reason for choosing the intermittent fast.

4.2 Deal with Hunger Pangs

It is no surprise that hunger is constant throughout intermittent fasting, and you may expect it to be far worse during regular fasting. This, however, is not always the case in practice. Hunger lasts around 20 mins, although most people are unaware of this since they do not wait to discover it. This book will provide you with practical suggestions for preventing hunger pains when fasting. Some individuals never experience true hunger since their appetite keeps them eating and staying satisfied constantly. True hunger is characterized by stomach grumbling and discomfort caused by the physical urge to consume food. While fasting, it is totally natural to experience hunger. The most difficult aspect is coming up with ideas for your next dinner. Hunger is a conditioned stimulus-response reaction that an individual may recondition.

What is the root cause of hunger?

Appetite is defined as the urge to consume food that is driven by hormones, senses, or feelings. When you are hungry, your hunger sends messages to your brain, but not all of these signals are beneficial to you. When you see something that looks delicious, your body may be led to hunger even after you've finished your meal. So, what is the source of hunger? Ghrelin, the hunger hormone, is responsible for the sensation of hunger. When your body is expecting a meal, it releases the hormone ghrelin. Ghrelin is mostly released by the stomach, although it is also released in minor amounts by the pancreas and small intestine. When the hormone is discharged into the circulation, it affects the hypothalamus, which is positioned below the eyes and under the midline of the cerebral cortex. A person will feel the desire to eat as a result of this. Food consumption may be increased by up to 30% due to the hormone cortisol. The first few days of your fast will be difficult since the want to eat will be continuous throughout the day. While fasting, you may experience hunger pains. Following are some ways to cope with these sensations while fasting.

How to Fight Hunger While Fasting: 8 Simple Steps

Because the body is used to regular meals, the system does not expect the change when you begin intermittent fasting. The urge to eat is associated with the reward system of the brain. Hunger may manifest itself not just on a physical level but also on a cognitive one. Keeping your appetite under control will allow you to maintain your fasting routine. Fortunately, there are a variety of strategies you may use to combat hunger when you are fasting.

Keep Yourself Hydrated: The body has a tendency to confuse the sensation of thirst with that of hunger. When you're hungry, you may be merely thirsty. Drinking water immediately after waking up will allow you to get a jump start on your hydration intake. Consume two to three liters of water every day, if at all possible. Staying hydrated helps you feel fuller for longer periods of time. However, excessive water consumption may cause valuable electrolytes to be flushed from the body, resulting in dehydration. Drinking lots of water is one of the most important tools you can use to keep your fast going. Approximately 30% of the water you consume comes from your diet. Therefore, you should account for this while fasting intermittently. To prevent eating and keep within your fasting objectives, you might add appetite suppressants to your water. If you find it difficult to drink plain sparkling water, you may add fasting vitamins to your drink to make it more bearable. Carbonated water is another one of the hacks that may be used when on a fast. In addition to having zero calories, it also includes carbon dioxide, which causes you to feel full when it fills your stomach. You may also take apple cider vinegar as a supplement while you're on an intermittent fasting schedule. Apple cider vinegar (ACV) provides several health advantages while also keeping your content without requiring you to break your fast. Taking apple cider vinegar in the morning or just before having a meal helps to absorb minerals from the meals you ate before the fast began. If you don't like the flavor of apple cider vinegar, try ACV gummies.

Get A Good Night's Sleep: Your appetite will be affected if you have irregular sleeping habits, are stressed, or use alcohol. It is important to go to bed and wake up early. Your blood sugar levels and hormones are also affected by poor sleep habits. These actions will cause hormone-induced hunger, prompting you to break your fast. You can control your hormone levels by getting adequate sleep, drinking less alcohol, and using stress-reduction tactics. For improved sleep quality, you need a comfortable and well-ventilated bedroom. It's also crucial to go to bed early and keep to a regular sleeping schedule in a peaceful setting. You should also avoid watching television before going to bed.

You should minimize your alcohol intake as much as possible before beginning your fasting phase. This stabilizes your blood sugar levels and reduces unpredictable hormones.

Fasting Hrs Should Be Scheduled Overnight: A 10–16-hour fast has been shown to induce the body to begin burning fat into energy from its stores, according to research. By releasing ketones into the body, promotes weight loss. It is a great way to get started with intermittent fasting. The fasting window is short, and one may eat the same number of calories every day. The ideal strategy to complete a 10–16-hour fast is to do it during your nocturnal sleeping hrs. For example, your eating schedule may be from 7 a.m. till 7 p.m. A mouse research found that time-restricted feeding protected mice against metabolic illnesses like diabetes and obesity, even when they ate the same number of calories as mice that ate anytime they wanted.

Consume Warm Liquids: Warm drinks, such as tea and coffee, assist your body to adjust to the fasting experience rapidly. According to research published by the National Center for Biotechnology Information, catechins (antioxidants found in tea) lower ghrelin release. A hot beverage fills the gaps left by eating by making you feel satisfied. Black coffee is healthy as long as it is served without milk or sugar. You should also avoid milk and sugar when drinking tea since they contain calories. You should be aware that some herbal teas include fruit sweeteners. It would be beneficial if you drank just zero-calorie green tea. If you're having trouble sticking to your intermittent fasting plan, consider bulletproof coffee, which is black coffee mixed with fats such as ghee, butter, or coconut oil. Healthy fats may aid in keeping you in ketosis. If you're a fasting purist, then, you should thoroughly avoid calories since even one more calorie will force you to break your fast.

Do a Little Exercising: When fasting, any kind of physical exercise is beneficial as long as it is done in moderation. Short bursts of activity can divert your attention away from eating. Walking, yoga, or Pilates are all fantastic ways to burn fat, build muscle, and tone down hunger sensations. When you play tennis, basketball, or football, it fools your mind into thinking you're not fasting. The brain concentrates on both exercise and activities. Walking works practically every muscle group in your body, increasing fat-burning potential. Walking helps your general health while also urging your body to burn fat for energy.

Distract Yourself: When we keep occupied on specific situations, it helps us cope with growing hunger levels. When our bodies anticipate a meal, we may feel hungry at meal times. You may keep yourself engaged by planning workouts or other things to keep you busy. Allowing boredom to sneak in will almost certainly lead to hunger. Because emotional hunger is linked to physical hunger, boredom leads to overeating. You may make an intermittent fasting strategy and schedule your time accordingly. You may start your day with some housework instead of breakfast. You may also schedule your work meetings around when you eat your lunch. Chewing gum is another strategy to distract yourself from hunger symptoms, but it should only be used as a last option. Sugar-free gum is the greatest alternative since it will not break your fast. Chewing gum momentarily relieves hunger, but it may cause you to get hungry again in the long term. As you come closer to your eating window, chewing gum is a good idea since the chewing sensation signals to your stomach that you'll be receiving food soon.

When you're not fasting, eat protein-rich, high-fat foods: Implementing a protein-rich and higher healthier fat diet is the greatest method to lay the groundwork for a low-carb diet. A high-fat, protein-rich diet can help you achieve your weight-loss objectives quicker. Between fasts, sticking to a protein-rich meal stabilizes blood sugar and makes you feel more satiated. You'll find that your intermittent fasting goes more easily, and you'll feel less hungry.

When you're not fasting, stay away from carbs: When you're not fasting, one of the diet modifications you should make is to reduce your carb consumption. Intermittent fasting isn't an excuse to consume low-quality food; rather, it's a strategy to make the most of your health and diet. Following a low-carbohydrate diet keeps you satisfied and your blood sugar in check. Sugary foods elevate blood glucose levels and induce insulin release, which triggers the secretion of hunger hormones even more. Carbs may be replaced with legumes, nutritious grains, and vegetables, which can keep you satisfied for a long time.

4.3 Practice Portion Control

Top nutritionists, dieters, and those attempting to try intermittent fasting all talk about portion management. Restaurants and other food establishments have distorted our perception of what is a portion of a main meal or snack. Furthermore, few individuals understand the need of portion control while dining out and at home. Many people assume that portion control equates to perpetual hunger, but this is not the case. Portion management does not mean that you should take just a few bites of everything on your plate. It entails consuming the quantity of food required by your body. Managing your meal amounts can help you discover you consume more than your body requires, whether you're on a fast or just want to start eating better.

Make mindful eating a habit: When you eat thoughtfully, you won't have that awful tummy sensation after a meal. It also helps you to appreciate the tastes and sensations that each item provides. It's difficult to concentrate only on your meal when there are so many distractions, such as cellphones with social networking platforms, computers with important tasks, and televisions with beloved movies. Eat slowly and thoroughly, chewing your meal well. You'll eat less and feel fuller without overeating this way. The issue is that it takes a long for your stomach to convey a message to your brain that it's full — generally 15 to 20 mins. Get up earlier in the morning to intentionally consume your breakfast, and take your time in the evening to really appreciate your supper. It's also been shown that mindful eating may help with bloating and stomach discomfort.

Switch plates: The more food on your plate, the bigger it is. Even if you just place a little amount of your food on it, your eye will send a signal to your brain and stomach that it's insufficient. Don't let this happen by replacing the dishes you've been using to serve your meals with smaller ones. That's the ruse restaurants employ to deceive us into ordering more, eating more, and spending more than we need to. They offer colossal dishes with a little quantity of food on them. You immediately assume it's too little for you and that you need to get more. If you're eating at home, use tiny plates and pile your food. This is the simplest approach to fool your eyes into thinking you're consuming a big amount of food. When dining out, request that your meal be served on tiny plates as well. It's what famous people do when they go out to eat.

Select treats that require peeling, shelling, or unwrapping: Pistachios, asparagus, oranges, grapefruit, kiwifruit, carrots, walnut and a variety of other foods that take some effort before eating are wonderful snack options. The length of time you spend peeling or shelling provides your stomach time to transmit a "satisfaction" signal to your brain, which helps you avoid overeating. Don't peel anything while preparing your lunch for work; save it for your lunch break.

Begin with a salad: This method works in both restaurants and at home. If you want to lose a lot of weight, you should try to cut down on bad fats as much as possible. Starting your meal with a container of low-calorie, high-greens salad will quell your appetite and cause you to consume less greasy meals. The same applies for desserts: before ordering your favorite pie, choose a fruit salad without dressings. Green salads are high in nutrients and antioxidants, which help you lose weight and feel and look better by reducing chronic stress, reducing inflammation, and enhancing vitality.

Avoid eating from a package or bag: If you carefully study a food label, you'll see information on how many calories and grams are in each serving. Take pretzels for example: 10 twists (about 60 grams) have roughly 230 calories. Consider how many twists are in each package and how many you consume in one sitting the same may be said for whole-wheat crisps or other diet-friendly treats found at the shop. Before you start eating, read the labels and calculate the portions and calories. Divide the contents of a box or bag into many pieces. Put them in little containers or zip-top bags and eat one anytime you're hungry. Use a kitchen scale to measure your food if there is no information regarding portions. It may seem absurd, but it's an easy method to figure out how many grams or oz. make up one serving.

Before a meal, drink a glass of water: When it comes to losing weight reduction, water is a fantastic weapon. It makes you feel filled faster and helps you avoid cravings. Not to mention that it provides you with extra energy, allowing you to work out more vigorously. A common suggestion is to drink a lot of water before each meal, but many people disregard it because they follow it incorrectly. The key is to drink plenty of water and wait at least 10 mins before eating. If you need to drastically reduce your calorie intake, drink water after each three spoons of food. When you're hungry, a glass of water can assist you figure out whether your body is craving food or if you're merely thirsty. Many individuals confuse thirst for hunger and eat when they really only need a glass of water.

Bring your meal to your pals to share: Restaurants tend to provide enormous quantities; so, why not reduce your calorie intake whilst saving money by sharing your food with family or friends? It's much better if they're also keeping track of their servings. If you don't have somebody to share your meal with, you might ask a server to bring you half a dish. Mindful eating is the key to portion management. It's all about eating for your health, not your waistline. It may take a long time and a lot of patience to figure out how to eat your proper meal quantity, but don't give up and allow space for errors.

Chapter 5: Breakfast Recipes For Intermittent Fasting

5.1 Fat Burning Green Smoothie
Prep Time: five mins
Cook Time: five mins
Servings: one
Ingredients

- one big ripe banana
- one cup roughly sliced mature kale
- 1 big ripe banana
- quarter ripe avocado
- one tbsp of chia seeds
- one cup vanilla unsweetened almond milk
- 2 tbsps of fresh honey
- 1 pound of ice cubes

Instructions

Mix the kale, banana, chia seeds, almond milk, avocado, and honey in a mixer. Mix on high till smooth and creamy. Mix in the ice till it is thoroughly smooth.

Nutrition Facts Fat 14.2g; Protein 5.9g; Sodium 198.9mg.

5.2 Low Carb Pancakes
Prep Time: 30 mins
Cook Time: twenty-five mins
Servings: 6
Ingredients

- 2 tsps baking powder
- quarter cup sugar-free applesauce
- one and a half cups whole-wheat flour
- 2 tsps melted coconut oil
- one tsp of sugar
- quarter tsp salt
- one and a half cups of unsweetened almond
- 1 tsp vanilla essence

Instructions

Mix flour, baking powder, and salt in a big mixing container. Mix the milk, applesauce, oil, sugar, and vanilla in a moderate mixing container. Make a well in the middle of the dry components and pour in the wet components, whisking till mixed. Allow the batter to settle for 10 to 15 mins without stirring. (The baking powder generates bubbles in the batter while it sits, resulting in fluffy pancakes). Cook over moderate heat in a big frypan or skillet covered with cooking spray. Using around quarter cup batter for each pancake, measure out pancakes and place them onto the pan without mixing the batter (or onto the grill). Cook for 2 to 4 mins, or till the edges are dry and bubbles appear on the top. Cook for another 2 to 4 mins on the other side till golden brown. Cook the rest of the batter in the same way, spraying the pan with cooking spray and lowering the heat as required.

Nutrition Facts Fat 8.42g; Protein 4.9g; Sodium 10mg

5.3 Keto Tumeric Milkshake
Prep Time: five mins
Cook Time: 5 mins
Servings: 1
Ingredients

- one sugar-free pellet
- half tsp cinnamon one sugar-free pellets
- one and a half cup coconut milk
- ice cubes as required
- 1 tsp turmeric
- salt as required
- half tsp coconut oil

Instructions

Mix turmeric, ginger, coconut milk, coconut oil, cinnamon, sugar-free pellets, and a bit of salt in a mixing jar. Mix all of the components in a thick milkshake. Pour into glasses and top with cinnamon powder. After that, grab a glass and pour the milkshake all the way to the top, then drizzle some cinnamon and turmeric on top. You may also throw in a couple of ice cubes just before serving.

Nutrition Facts Fat; 35g, Protein; 1.6g,

5.4 Breakfast Burritos
Prep Time: thirty-five mins
Cook Time: twenty-five mins
Servings: 6
Ingredients

- 10 flour tortillas
- 1 (16 oz.) can of refried beans
- 1-pound bacon
- 10 eggs
- 8 oz. shredded Cheddar cheese

Instructions

In a big, deep-pan, cook the bacon. Cook till uniformly browned over moderate-high heat. Drain the water and put it aside. Prepare the tortillas by wrapping them in foil and placing them in the oven. In an oiled skillet, fry the eggs till hard. Heat the refried beans in a small saucepan. Refried beans, 2 slices of bacon, 1 egg, and a little cheese go on top of each tortilla. Serve burritos made with tortillas.

Nutrition Facts Fat 39.1g; Protein 25.6g Sodium; 1180.9mg.

5.5 Fat-Burning Coconut Cookies

Prep Time: 35 mins
Cook Time: twenty-five mins
Servings: six

Ingredients

- quarter cup almond flour
- ¾ cup granular sucralose sweetener
- 3 eggs
- 1 tsp almond milk
- half cup butter
- half tbsp heavy cream
- 1 tsp almond milk
- half cup unsweetened coconut flakes
- 6 tbsps coconut flour
- quarter cup almond flour
- one tsp baking powder

Instructions

Preheat the oven to 350°F (180°C) (175 degrees C). Using parchment paper, line a baking sheet. In a mixing container, cream together the sweetener and butter. Mix the eggs, almond milk, and heavy cream in a mixing container and whisk till smooth. With a spoon, scrape down the sides. Mix baking powder, coconut flakes, baking soda, coconut flour, almond flour, and salt in a separate dish. Mix in the butter till the dough comes together. Using a tsp, drop cookie batter onto baking sheets. Bake for 17 mins in a pre-heated oven till golden brown. Cool for 3 mins on the baking sheet before transporting it to a wire rack to cool thoroughly.

Nutrition Facts Fat 8.9g; Protein 2g; Sodium 210.9mg

5.6 Spinach Frittata

Prep Time: twenty mins
Cook Time: 10 mins
Servings: 4

Ingredients

- 2 tbsps extra virgin olive oil
- one-eighth tsp freshly ground pepper
- 2 tbsps sliced sun-dried tomatoes, optional
- 1 big clove of garlic, crushed
- quarter tsp salt

- 2 oz. (56g) of goat cheese
- one-third cup (about 1 ounce, 30g) grated Parmesan cheese
- 8 oz. (225g) or more fresh sliced spinach (or use baby spinach)
- 9 big eggs
- 1 moderate onion, sliced (about 1 cup)
- 2 tbsps milk

Instructions

Whisk milk, eggs, & Parmesan cheese in a mixing dish. Add the pepper and salt and mix well. Remove from the equation. Heat the olive oil over moderate heat in an ovenproof, nonstick skillet. Add the onion, then cook for 4 to 5 mins, or till transparent. Cook for another minute after adding the garlic and sun-dried tomatoes (if using). A handful of spinach at a time should be added. Toss in the onion with tongs. Add additional spinach to the pan when the fresh spinach starts to wilt and create space in the pan. Spread the spinach mixture evenly over the bottom of the pan after it has wilted. The onion and spinach pour the egg mixture. Lift the mixture along the pan's sides with a spoon to allow the egg mixture to flow below. Over the top of the frittata mixture, drizzle goat cheese chunks. Reduce to a low heat setting, then cover the pan. Cook for 10 to 13 mins on the stovetop, or till everything except the center of the frittata is done. (You may need to check the frittata a few times to see how it's setting.) The wavy center should remain. Preheat the oven to broil. Place the baking dish in the oven's top third. Broil for 3 mins, or till golden brown on top. Remove using oven mitts and set aside to cool for a few mins. To serve, cut into wedges.

Nutrition Facts Fat 21; Protein 23; Sodium 520mg;

5.7 Low-Calorie Porridge
Prep Time: 3 mins   Cook Time: 7 mins   Servings: 3
Ingredients

- Berries
- Almond paste
- 50 g oat flakes
- 130 ml water
- 1 tweak of of salt

Instructions

Make the water hot in a kettle. In a container, mix the oat flakes and a touch of salt. Fill the basin halfway with hot water. Mix the porridge thoroughly till it has a creamy consistency. Assemble your toppings and place them on top of the porridge.

Nutrition Facts Fat 0.0g; Protein 2.6; Sodium 52.2mg

Chapter 6: Lunch Recipes For Intermittent Fasting

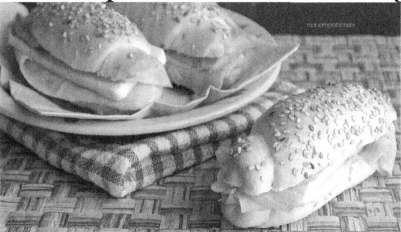

6.1 Jars of Chicken Spring Rolls

Prep Time: 35 mins   Cook Time: 20 mins   Servings: 8

Ingredients

- 1-quart oil for deep frying

- 1 small carrot, grated

- quarter cup barbeque sauce

- 1 dash of soy sauce

- 1 (14 oz.) package spring roll wrappers

- 1 small onion, grated

- 2 (10 oz.) can chunk chicken, drained and flaked

- 1 dash of hot pepper sauce

- 1 dash Worcestershire sauce

- half cup finely shredded cabbage

Instructions

Heat the oil to 375 degrees F in a deep-fryer or a big, heavy saucepan (190 degrees C). Mix the onion, carrot, chicken, hot pepper sauce, barbeque sauce, hot pepper sauce, soy sauce, and Worcestershire sauce in a moderate mixing container. 1 spoonful of the chicken combination should be placed in the middle of each spring roll wrapper. Wet your fingers and the edges of the wrapper with water. Roll the filling around with your hands. Seams should be pressed together to seal them. Deep fry the spring rolls in small batches for 4 mins, or till golden brown. Using paper towels, absorb any excess liquid.

Nutrition Facts Fat 13.9g; Protein 16.2g; Sodium 586.8mg

6.2 Zucchini Noodle Casserole

Prep Time: 20 mins   Cook Time: 40 mins   Servings: 4

Ingredients

- 5 zucchini squash, cut into the shape of noodles

- 3 tbsps olive oil
- salt and black pepper
- half cup shredded mozzarella cheese
- 1 (7 oz.) Greek yogurt
- 18 ounce) jar marinara sauce
- as required crushed garlic
- 1 tweak of of Italian seasoning
- half cup shredded mozzarella cheese

Instructions

Preheat the oven to 400 degrees Fahrenheit (200 degrees C). In a big skillet, heat 1 oil over moderate-high heat. In batches, cook enough zucchini to fill the pan with 1 tbsp of garlic till softened and slightly browned, 5 to 7 mins. Using the rest of the zucchini, oil and garlic, repeat the process. Fill a baking dish halfway with the cooked zucchini mixture. In a saucepan over low heat, whisk together marinara sauce, yogurt, Italian seasoning, salt, and black pepper; simmer and stir till sauce is warm through, 3 to 5 mins. In the baking dish, pour the sauce over the zucchini mixture. Over the top, add mozzarella and a touch of Italian spice. Cook for 15 to 25 mins in a warmed up oven till the cheese is melted.

Nutrition Facts Fat 17.7g; Protein 12g; Sodium 620.1mg.

6.3 Fish Tacos

Prep Time: 20 mins   Cook Time: 40 mins   Servings: 4

Ingredients

- cups shredded cabbage
- half cup salsa
- 1 tsps salt
- 3 lbs. fillets of tilapia
- 1 tsp chipotle peppers
- 1 tomato, sliced
- 16 (5 inches) corn tortillas
- 1 tbsp. black pepper
- 1 avocado - sliced
- 1 half tbsp fresh cilantro (sliced)
- 2 cups of shredded cheese
- cooking spray
- A tsp of paprika
- 2 onions (sliced)
- half cup plain fat-free yogurt
- 2 tbsps lime juice

- 1 tbsp garlic powder

Instructions

Season tilapia fillets with salt, garlic powder, black pepper and paprika after rubbing them with 2 tbsp of lime juice. Using cooking spray, coat both sides of the fillet. Preheat the grill to moderate heat and brush the grate gently with oil. In a mixer, mix the yogurt, 2 tbsp cilantro, lime juice and chipotle pepper; pulse till thoroughly mixd. Set aside. Grill tilapia till it can easily be split using a fork, approximately 6 mins on a separate side, on a hot grill. In a pan over low heat, cook each corn tortilla for approximately 1 minute. Serve grilled fish with cabbage lime sauce, cheese, salsa, tomato, avocado, and onions on corn tortillas.

Nutrition Facts Fat 11g; Protein 31.5g; Sodium 846.7mg

6.4 Lemon Green Beans

Prep time: 5 mins
Cook time: 25 mins

Serving: 6

Ingredients

- 1 pound fresh green beans, rinsed and trimmed
- quarter cup sliced almonds
- 2 tsps lemon pepper
- 2 tbsp butter

Instructions

In a steamer, place green beans over 1 inch of boiling water. Cook and cover for approximately 10 mins till it's tender and still firm; drain. Meanwhile, in a pan over moderate heat, melt the butter. Toast the almonds in a skillet, and season with lemon pepper for taste. Toss in the green beans well enough to coat.

Nutrition Facts Fat 5.9g; Protein 2.3g; Sodium 185.8mg

6.5 Eggplant Parmesan Panini

Prep time: 25 mins

Cook time: 45 mins

Serving: 8

Ingredients

- half cup sliced fresh basil
- 8 tbsps olive oil
- 8 oz. ricotta cheese
- 1 half tbsps salt
- 4 cups pasta sauce
- 1 eggplant, cut into 3/4 inch slices
- 6 oz. shredded mozzarella cheese

- half cup grated Parmesan cheese
- 1 egg, beaten

Instructions

Season the eggplant slices on both sides with salt. Place the slices in a sieve with a dish below to catch the liquid that will evaporate as the eggplant sweats. Allow for 30 mins of resting time. Preheat the oven to 350 °F (175 degrees C). Mix the ricotta, mozzarella, and quarter cup Parmesan cheese in a moderate mixing basin. Mix the egg and basil in a mixing container. Rinse the eggplant well in cold water to eliminate any salt. 4 tbsps olive oil, heated in a big pan over moderate heat brown from each side about one layer of eggplant in the pan. Repeat with the rest of the eggplant slices, using more oil as needed. 1 half cups spaghetti sauce, distributed evenly in a 9x13 inch baking dish. On top of the sauce, arrange a layer of eggplant slices. half of the cheese mixture should be placed on top of the eggplant. Continue stacking till all of the eggplant and cheese mixtures has been used. Add the rest of the sauce over the layers, then top with the leftover Parmesan cheese. Bake for 30 to 45 mins, till the sauce, is bubbling, in a warmed up oven.

Nutrition Fact Fat 17.1g; Protein 15g; Sodium 671.6mg

6.6 Paleo Chicken Stew

Prep Time: 15 mins   Cook Time: 35 mins   Servings: 6

Ingredients

- 1 cup fresh spinach, or as required
- 1 small red onion, sliced
- 1 tweak of paprika, or more as required
- sea salt as required
- 1 tweak of crushed red pepper, or more as required
- 2 tsps olive oil
- 2 skinless, boneless chicken breast halves, cut into cubes
- 2 sweet potatoes, skinned and sliced
- half cup chicken broth, or more as required
- 2 cloves garlic, crushed

Instructions

In a saucepan, heat the olive oil over moderate-high heat. 5 mins in high oil, sauté onion and garlic till softened. Mix the sweet potatoes, chicken, spinach, paprika, crushed red pepper, and sea salt with onion and garlic in a saucepan. Pour chicken stock into the pot to make the mixture soupy or stew. Bring the stock to a boil, then lower to moderate-low heat and cook for 30 mins, or till the chicken is just no longer pink inside the center and the potatoes are soft.

Nutrition Facts Fat 2.6g; Protein 9.6g; Sodium 223mg

6.7 Chicken Salad with Walnuts and Grapes

Prep Time: 25 mins   Cook Time: 25 mins   Servings: 4

Ingredients

- 1 half tbsp and half tsp mayonnaise
- ⅔ Granny Smith apples, cut into small chunks
- 1 half tbsp and half tsp creamy salad dressing
- ⅔ cup sliced walnuts, or as required
- 1 stalks celery, sliced
- 1 tbsp lemon juice
- 2 half tbsps and half tsp vanilla yogurt
- 1 ⅓ cooked chicken breasts, shredded
- 1 red onion, sliced
- 8 ⅓ seedless red grapes, halved

Instructions

1.   Mix the apple chunks, red onion, walnuts, shredded chicken, celery, and lemon juice in a big mixing container.

2.   Mix the vanilla yogurt, salad dressing, and mayonnaise; pour over the chicken mix and swirl to coat.

3.   Toss fresh grapes into the mix gently.

Nutrition Facts Fat 22.7g; Protein 17.7g; Sodium 127.5mg

Chapter 7: Dinner Recipes For Intermittent Fasting

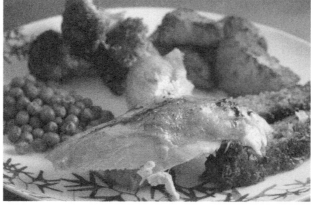

7.1 Honey Sesame Salmon

Prep Time: 20 mins　　　　　Cook Time: 20 mins　　　　　Servings: 2

Ingredients

- Pepper, for sprinkling
- Salt, for sprinkling
- 1-pound salmon fillets
- quarter cup water
- 2 tbsps of sesame oil
- quarter cup honey
- 2 tbsps of soy sauce
- 2 cloves garlic, crushed
- juice of 1 lemon
- half tsp Cornstarch, dissolved

Instructions

Preheat the oven to 375 degrees F. Season the salmon with salt and pepper before baking it for 20 mins (cook time will depside on fillet size). Meanwhile, add water, lemon, honey, sesame oil, soy sauce, and garlic to a saucepan. Bring the water to a boil. Cook till the cornstarch mixture has thickened. Serve the sauce with the fish.

Nutrition Facts Fat 13.2 g; Protein 31.7 g; Sodium 446.7 mg

7.2 Chicken with Cauliflower Rice Casserole

Prep Time: 60 mins　　　　　Cook Time: 25 mins　　　　　Servings: 2

Ingredients

- 3 cups shredded cooked chicken breast
- quarter tsp cayenne pepper
- 2 tsps garlic powder
- half tsp ground pepper

- 6 oz. cream cheese, softened
- quarter tsp salt
- 1 (12-ounce) package of riced cauliflower
- half cup scallions
- 1 tsp dry mustard
- 1 tsp dried oregano
- 1 tsp onion powder
- 1 half cups shredded Cheddar cheese

Instructions

Preheat the oven to 400 degrees Fahrenheit. Using cooking spray, cover a baking dish. In a microwave-safe container, place the cauliflower. Cover closely and heat on high for 4 mins, or till tender. In a big mixing container, mix garlic powder, cream cheese, oregano, mustard, pepper, onion powder, salt, cayenne, and 14 cup scallions; mix with an electric mixer on moderate speed 1 minute, or till smooth. Mix the cauliflower, chicken, and 1 cup of Cheddar cheese in a mixing container. Fill the baking dish halfway with the mixture. Cover with foil and top with the rest of the 12 cups of Cheddar. Bake for 30 mins or till bubbling. Uncover and bake for another 10 mins, or till the cheese is golden brown. Remove the pan from the oven and top with the rest of the 14 cup scallions. Allow for a 10-minute rest period before serving.

Nutrition Facts Fat 13g; Protein 32g; Sodium 439mg;

7.3 Lentil and Vegetable Curry
Prep Time: 60 mins   Cook Time: 25 mins   Servings: 2
Ingredients

- 300g (1 small) eggplant, cut into 2.5cm dice
- 1 tbsp olive oil
- 3/4 cup dried French-style lentils
- 1 big onion, thinly sliced
- 400g (half moderate) cauliflower, cut into small florets
- half cup reduced-fat plain yogurt, to serve
- half reduced-salt vegetable stock cube, crumbled
- 150g green beans, topped, halved
- 400g can no added salt sliced tomatoes
- 2 tbsps korma paste
- 100g button mushrooms, halved
- 2 garlic cloves, crushed
- half cup sliced coriander
- 2 half cups of water

- 2 small whole meal pita bread, halved, to serve

Instructions

Heat the oil in a big, deep nonstick frying pan or a big deep saucepan at moderate heat. Cook, often tossing, for 3-4 mins, or when the onion and garlic you've added are tender and light golden in color. Mix the korma paste and lentils in a mixing container. Cook for 1 minute, stirring constantly. Add the tomatoes, water, and stock cube to a mixing container. Put the water to a boil. Lower the heat, cover with the lid and cook for 10 mins. Mix the cauliflower, eggplant, and mushrooms in a container and mix. Cook for 15 mins with the lid on. Add the beans and mix well. Simmer for another 5 mins, uncovered, or till veggies are soft. Remove the pan from the heat. Add the coriander and mix well. Serve with pita bread and yogurt.

Nutrition Facts Fat 4.2g; Protein 6.2g; Sodium 416mg;

7.4 Honey Garlic Shrimp

Prep Time: 15 mins   Cook Time: 5 mins   Servings: 4

Ingredients

- 1 lb. moderate shrimp
- quarter cup of soy sauce
- 3 tsps olive oil
- sliced green onion
- one-third cup of honey
- 2 garlic cloves, crushed
- 1 tsp crushed ginger

Instructions

Mix the honey, soy sauce, garlic, and ginger in a moderate mixing container. Half will be used for the marinade, and the other half will be used to cook the shrimp. Put the shrimp in a big sealable container or a bag. Pour half of the marinade/sauce mixture on top, give it a good shake or mix, and let the shrimp marinate for 15 mins or up to 8 hrs in the refrigerator. The rest of the marinade should be covered and kept refrigerated. In a pan, heat the olive oil over moderate-high heat. In a skillet, place the shrimp. (Remove the used marinade) Cook for 45 seconds on one side, then flip to cook for another 45 seconds. Pour in the rest of the marinade/sauce and simmer till the shrimp is fully cooked, approximately 1-2 mins longer. Serve the shrimp with the prepared marinade sauce and a green onion garnish on brown rice with steamed veggies on the side.

Nutrition Facts Fat 3.8g; Protein 28.7g; Sodium 1,118.9mg

7.5 Turkey Meatball and Kale Soup

Prep Time: 5 mins   Cook Time: 15 mins   Servings: 2

Ingredients

- half lb. ground turkey
- Olive oil

- Bone broth for the soup
- 1 flax egg
- quarter cup almond flour

Instructions

In a moderate mixing container, mix all of the components and add season as required. Sear in olive oil in a moderate saucepan, but don't cook all the way through. When the meat is boiling in the broth, it will continue to cook. Cook with crushed garlic, salt and pepper, red pepper flakes, and Italian seasoning in your favorite bone broth. Add the carrots, 2 handfuls of sliced kale, and the turkey meatballs after the liquid has reached a steady boil. Reduce heat to low and cook for 10 mins. And then serve.

Nutrition Facts Fat 6.0g; Protein 14.8g; Sodium 110.2mg;

7.6 Chicken Provolone

Prep Time: five mins   Cook Time: 25 mins   Servings: four

Ingredients

- four slices provolone cheese
- quarter tsp pepper
- 4 thin slices prosciutto or deli ham
- Butter-flavored cooking spray
- 8 fresh basil leaves
- four boneless skinless chicken breast halves (4 oz. each)

Instructions

1. Season the chicken with salt and pepper.

2. Cook chicken in a big pan sprayed with cooking spray till the thermometer reaches 165 °, about 4-5 mins on each side.

3. Top with basil, prosciutto, and cheese on an ungreased baking sheet.

4. Broil 6-8 inches from the flame for one to two mins, or till cheese is dissolved.

Nutrition Facts Fat 6g; Protein 33g; Sodium 435mg

7.7 Spaghetti Diablo with Shrimp

Prep Time: five mins   Cook Time: 25 mins   Servings: four

Ingredients

- half tsp olive oil
- half onion, sliced
- one can of diced tomatoes
- quarter cup white wine
- 6 oz. cooked shrimp
- salt and ground black pepper

- half green bell pepper, sliced
- quarter cup grated Pecorino-Romano cheese
- half yellow bell pepper, sliced
- 4 oz.' spaghetti
- quarter tsp dried oregano
- three cloves garlic, crushed
- quarter tsp red pepper flakes
- quarter cup sliced fresh parsley, divided
- quarter tsp dried basil

Instructions

1.   In a Dutch oven, warm the oil across moderate-high flame. 5 to 7 mins in heated oil, stir and cook yellow bell pepper, green bell pepper, onions, and garlic till tender.

2.   Season with salt & pepper.

3.   Bring the bell pepper combination to a boil with the tomatoes, alcohol, quarter cup parsley, oregano, basil and red pepper flakes; lower heat to low and cover the Dutch oven.

4.   Cook, stirring regularly, for approximately 2 hrs, or till the tomatoes have broken down.

5.   Bring a big saucepan of water to a boil, lightly salted. Cook spaghetti in boiling water for approximately 10 mins.

6.   Cook, occasionally stirring, till the drained pasta and shrimp are fully cooked but still stiff to the touch, 2 to 4 mins longer.

7.   Toss with the rest of the Pecorino-Romano cheese and parsley before serving.

Nutrition Facts Fat 3.5g; Protein 29g; Sodium 233mg

Chapter 8: Dessert Recipes For Intermittent Fasting

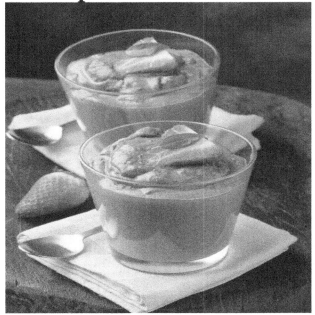

8.1 Citrus Dark Chocolate Mousse

Prep Time: five mins
Cook Time: fifteen mins
Servings: 5

Ingredients

- one tsp of brewed coffee
- 85g of dark chocolate
- one tweak of of rock salt
- one tsp of orange zest
- half tsp of lime zest
- 3 moderate eggs

Instructions

In a small dish, mix orange and lime zest. On top of the double boiler, mix the chocolate and coffee with the zest over warm water. To keep the mixture from bubbling, stir it. Remove the chocolate from the heat after it has melted and put it away to cool. The egg whites and salt should be whisked together. Stir the egg yolks in the chocolate mixture, then pour the mixture over the egg whites and gently fold them in. Make small containers or glasses out of the mixture. Refrigerate for around four hrs prior to serving.

Nutrition Facts Fat 36g; Protein 10g; Sodium 294mg;

8.2 Peanut Butter Cookies

Prep Time: fifteen mins
Cook Time: 10 mins
Servings: 24

Ingredients

- half tsp salt
- 2 big eggs
- one and a half tsps baking soda
- one cup crunchy peanut butter
- one cup unsalted butter
- one tsp baking powder
- one cup white sugar
- two and a half cups all-purpose flour
- one cup packed brown sugar

Instructions

In a mixing container, mix together cream butter, peanut butter, and sugar; include in the eggs. Combine flour, baking powder, baking soda, and salt in a separate dish, then add the butter mixture. Refrigerate the dough for 1 hour. Make 1 inch balls out of the dough and place them on baking pans. Using a fork, flatten each ball into a crisscross pattern. Bake for approximately 10 mins in a warm uped 375°F oven till the cookies appear brown.

Nutrition Facts Fat 136g; Protein 4.5g; Sodium 209.4mg

8.3 Fruit Salad

Prep Time: five mins
Cook Time: twenty mins
Servings: eight

Ingredients

- four kiwis
- one cocktail strawberries
- 20 oz. of can pineapple chunks
- 2 apples
- 2 bananas
- 1 can of peach pie filling

Instructions

Toss the diced apples with the leftover pineapple juice in a small container. Allow resting for 7 to 10 mins. Mix the peach pie and pineapple pieces in a big salad dish. Remove the apples from the pineapple juice and mix them with the pie filling and pineapple mixture in a mixing container. Let seven to ten mins for the sliced bananas to soak up the saved pineapple juice. Peel and slice the kiwifruit, as well as half of the strawberries. Set aside the rest of the half of the strawberries. Remove the bananas from the pineapple juice and stir them into the pie filling. Toss in the strawberries that have been cut. Arrange kiwi slices and strawberry slices around the edges of the serving basin. Chill before serving.

Nutrition Facts Fat 0.5g; Protein 2.1g; Sodium 15mg;

8.1 Grapefruit Meringue Nests with Mixed Berries

Prep Time: 25 mins
Cook Time: one hr thirty mins
Servings: 8

Ingredients

Meringue Nests

- one tsp grapefruit peel
- half cup sugar
- four egg whites
- one-eighth tsp cream of tartar

Berries

- 4 oz. of raspberries
- quarter cup sugar
- 2 lbs. strawberries
- 4 oz. of blueberries
- quarter cup of grapefruit juice

Instructions

Meringues: Preheat the oven to 200 °F. Use parchment paper to line a big cookie sheet. In a big mixer, mix egg whites and cream. Drizzle in sugar 2 tbsp, beating till sugar dissolves, and meringue stands in stiff, creamy peaks. Gently mix grapefruit peel into a meringue. On a prepared sheet, divide the mixture into even mounds and spaced approximately 3 inches apart. Form mounds into 3-inch circular nests by pressing the back of a spoon into the center of each meringue. Bake for 2 hrs till firm. Turn off the oven and let the meringues in there to dry for 2 hrs or overnight. Remove the parchment gently after it has dried. Meringues may be kept at room temperature for around 2 weeks.

Berries: Mix blueberries, raspberries, and half of the strawberries in a big mixing container. Add sugar and grapefruit juice to a 12-inch skillet. On moderate heat to boiling, stir now and then Boil for two mins, or till the sugar has dissolved and the syrup has turned a clear pink color. Cook for 1-3 mins, or till the first half of the strawberries have released their juices and softened. In a big mixing basin, pour the mixture over the uncooked berries. Stir slowly till everything is fully mixed. Place the nests of meringue on serving plates. Spread berries among the nests and drizzle with grapefruit syrup. Serve right away.

Nutrition Facts Fat 40g; Protein 20g; Sodium 400mg;

8.5 Mango and Passionfruit Roulade

Prep Time: twenty mins
Cook Time: fifteen mins
Servings: four

Ingredients

- 85g sugar
- 3 eggs

- 250g of frozen raspberries
- 1 tsp of vanilla extract
- One tub of Greek yogurt
- 2 mangoes
- 85g plain flour, sifted
- one tsp baking powder
- one tbsp of sugar
- two ripe passion fruits

Instructions

Warm up the oven to 180°C. In a big mixing container, combine the eggs and sugar till it's thick and light. After that, wrap in the flour and baking powder, followed by the vanilla. Place the mixture in the pan, tilting it to level it out, and bake for fourteen to fifteen mins till it's brown. Place on a new piece of paper that has been powdered with 1 tbsp caster sugar. Allow cooling fully after rolling the paper within the sponge. Fold the sugar, passion fruit pulp, and one-third of the mango and raspberries. Unroll the sponge, spread with filling, then roll-up.

Nutrition Facts Fat 3g; Protein 5g; Sodium 256mg;

8.6 Strawberry-Chocolate Greek Yogurt

Prep Time: ten mins
Cook Time: 180 mins
Servings: 32

Ingredients

- one cup of sliced strawberries
- two tbsp. honey
- quarter cup of chocolate chips
- 3 cups plain Greek yogurt
- one tsp vanilla extract

Instructions

Using parchment paper, line in a baking sheet. Mix the yogurt, honey, and vanilla extract in a moderate mixing container. Make a rectangle on the lined baking sheet. Drizzle the chocolate chips on top and spread the strawberries on top. Freeze for at least three hrs, or till extremely firm. Slice to pieces to serve.

Nutrition Facts Fat 1.3g; Protein 2g; Sodium 7.6mg

8.7 Almond Butter Chocolate Chip Cookies

Prep Time: 15 mins
Cook Time: 35 mins
Servings: fifteen

Ingredients

- quarter cup sliced peanuts

- one egg
- 1 cup of almond butter
- half cup of chocolate chips
- 1 tsp of baking soda
- half cup of brown sugar

Instructions

Warm up the oven to 350°F. Line two baking pans with parchment paper. In a moderate mixing container, whisk together the egg. Mix almond butter, brown sugar, and baking soda in a mixing container and whisk till smooth.Mix peanuts and chocolate chips in a mixing container. To create each cookie, take roughly 1 tbsp of dough and roll it into a compact ball. Place the cookies 1 inch apart on the prepared pan pans. With the tip of a spoon, gently push down on each ball. Bake the cookies for 9 to 10 mins, or till the tops are cracked, and the edges are brown. Allow cooling for 10 mins on the pan.

Nutrition Facts Fat 10g; Protein 4g; Sodium 108mg

Conclusion

In conclusion, intermittent fasting has indeed been scientifically proven to be a pleasant and effective way to lose weight and get favorable health advantages for women over 60. Intermittent fasting is a method of allowing the body to metabolize the food it has consumed. On the other hand, scientists have discovered that this fasting approach is not suited for everyone. As a result, it's a good idea to get medical advice before fasting. Intermittent fasting side effects are caused by the body's inability to adjust to the new eating schedule. As one continues to fast, the body will get used to it, and the negative effects will disappear. Intermittent fasting should also be avoided if one has a history of health problems, such as high blood pressure. Intermittent fasting is a fantastic alternative to difficult-to-maintain fad diets for women over 60. Time-restricted eating allows women to lose weight without limiting their calorie intake or depriving themselves of essential nutrients. Intermittent fasting may easily be incorporated into everyday activities as part of a well-balanced diet. It is a kind of eating that alternates between eating and fasting intervals. Intermittent fasting may be done in a variety of ways, including twice-weekly, alternate-day, and time-restricted.

Intermittent fasting has various effects on women. Women should be aware of potential dangers to their reproductive health, bone health, and general well-being. Whereas with disadvantages, there are certain advantages like weight reduction, diabetes prevention, and improved heart health are all potential health advantages of intermittent fasting, according to evidence.

While fasting, understanding how one reacts to various meals might assist in eating in a beneficial manner for metabolic health. There are a few things one can do to maximize the health advantages of intermittent fasting. Using a notebook to keep track of the routine may help to notice improvement and motivate one to exercise, prevent snacking, and eat at the right times. It may also urge one to develop a fasting habit or lifestyle.

When fasting, it's also beneficial to remain aware. Take time to exercise and re-energize the body to remain active and on track with one's dietary cycles. This may help one to get the most out of the workouts, avoid weight gain, and keep track of the food intake.

Making an intermittent fasting schedule will assist in being active and adhering to a fasting lifestyle. It has a plethora of health advantages that may last a lifetime. If fasting is safe for you, it is well worth it to gain the many health advantages of intermittent fasting.

ANTI-INFLAMMATORY DIET COOKBOOK FOR BEGINNERS

Introduction

Inflammation is a medical term that describes an increase in size in a specific region of the body. Typically, a painful, crimson, and hot sensation may be felt in the region that is inflamed. It is possible for it to manifest in any portion of the body when an illness or damage is present. The symptoms that were stated before are typical, with inflammation that lasts just a brief time. Inflammation that lasts for an extended period of time, also known as chronic irritation, is the form of inflammation that is responsible for the development of illness. The inflammatory response is among the defense mechanisms that your body uses to keep itself healthy. In addition to that, it helps the body fight against diseases. Inflammation is generally considered to be beneficial since it plays a significant role in the amazing healing process that occurs inside the body. There is also a subset of the population that suffers from a form of the medical disease that prevents their immune systems from operating as well as they should. This illness may result in irritation of a low level or for a short period of time, but it also has the potential to cause inflammation that lasts for a prolonged period of time or is chronic. Infections and other disorders may also lead to a condition known as chronic inflammation, which can affect almost any part of the body. It is possible to have this symptom if you suffer from psoriasis, asthma, rheumatoid arthritis, or any of a number of other illnesses. According to the findings of several studies, persistent inflammation may possibly have a role in the development of cancer. In addition to these disorders, there is growing evidence in the medical literature that the foods we eat may also have a role in the development of continuous inflammation. That being said, modifying your eating routine in any way will be of great assistance to you in the event that you are afflicted with inflammation of any kind.

Symptoms of an inflammatory response

The following is a list of some of the indicators that you may be experiencing irritation in any part of your body:

- Bloating around the abdomen
- Achy joints
- Loss of appetite
- Acid reflux
- Nausea
- Diarrhea, Gas
- Cramping

If you encounter any of these signs, then you need to make an appointment with your primary care physician as soon as possible. They will be able to assist you in determining whether or not you are indeed suffering from irritation or if the signs you are feeling are those of another ailment. The great news is that just by making simple adjustments to your diet, you may gradually bring down inflammation levels in your body in a natural way. It is the method that emphasizes moderate but consistent progress toward better health over the long term. You are able to do this by following a diet that reduces inflammation.

CHAPTER 1: What exactly is meant by the term "anti-inflammatory diet"?

Actually, there is no such thing as a diet that is guaranteed to reduce inflammation for any particular health condition, arthritis included, of course. There is more than one kind of diet designed to reduce inflammation. Diets such as the Dietary Pattern and the diet recommended by Dr. Weil are both examples of diets that can reduce inflammation. These dietary plans emphasize the consumption of foods that either contribute to irritation in the body or work to alleviate it. Diets designed to lower inflammation will naturally include products and foods known for their anti-inflammatory properties. In addition to this, it forbids the eating of items that promote inflammation. Antioxidants may be found in abundance in a wide variety of plant-based meals. Antioxidants, according to the findings of multiple research, may neutralize the effects of free agents in the body. When free radicals gather in big enough numbers, they may cause harm to the cells of the body. Because of this, any diet designed to reduce inflammation includes a substantial amount of food high in antioxidants. These kinds of diets have as their primary objective the internal cleaning and maintenance of the body as a whole. Your immune system will mend, and your digestion will become better if you follow this diet.

Different kinds of anti-inflammatory foods to eat

There are many well-known dietary treatments available today that can reduce inflammation. Diets such as the Mediterranean Diet, DASH Diet, and the Anti-Inflammatory Diet developed by Dr. Weil are all examples of diets that help reduce inflammation. In the subsequent chapters, we will discuss these various dietary plans.

Foods that are known to trigger inflammation

Inflammation might be caused by both the ways in which we eat and the items that we consume. You may get a head start on your journey toward an anti-inflammatory diet by avoiding foods that cause inflammation. This is just one of the methods by that you can get started.

These foods may be classified into one of the following six categories:

- Vegetable Oils (Includes Seed Oils)
- High Fructose and Sugary Foods
- Excess Alcohol
- Artificial Trans Fats
- Refined Carbs
- Processed Meat

Vegetable Oils (Includes Seed Oils)

A significant amount of omega-6 oils may be found in these oils. In spite of the fact that they are required by the body, they are responsible for an increase in irritation if there is a greater proportion of omega-six to omega-three inside the body. During the 20th century, people consumed around 130% more vegetable oils than they did in the previous century on average. According to the opinions of several experts, it is one of the factors that contributes to the rising incidence of inflammatory-related health disorders. According to the findings of these studies, excessive use of these oils might lead to inflammation. It is important to keep in mind that vegetable oils may be utilized in cooking and can also be found as an ingredient in a variety of processed meals. You should cut down on your consumption of vegetable oils to either forestall the development of irritation in the body or bring about a reduction in its severity.

High Fructose and Sugary Foods

Foods that are high in glucose and foods that have a significant amount of fructose should be at the top of your list of foods to steer clear of. There are two primary offenders in the food that we follow on a daily basis that is responsible for inflammation. In the first place, we have high fructose corn syrup, and in the second place, we have regular sugar. These seem to be the two most frequent kinds of sugar that are consumed in today's diets all across the world. According to the findings of one research, the body sustains a significant amount of harm as a direct result of the consumption of these added sugars. However, fructose and all of the other forms of sugars that you discover naturally occurring in all of our meals are not inherently harmful or sinful in and of themselves. They are genuinely beneficial since they provide the body with the much-required energy. The problem is when you take in too much information, which may happen very rapidly. Simply consuming a huge can of Coke would provide you with the same amount of glucose that your body requires for the whole of one week in a single session. However, do you just drink a single can of soda at a time? There are some folks who consume at least three sodas every day. A diet that is heavy in sugar may increase the risk of developing breast cancer, according to the findings of another research. Sugar may also be found in the form of sucrose. In addition, there is evidence to indicate that consuming meals high in sugar may inhibit or counteract the anti-inflammatory benefits of omega-three fatty acids. Excessive consumption of fructose has been associated with an increased risk of developing chronic illnesses such as cancer, diabetes, fatty liver disease, insulin resistance, chronic kidney disease, and obesity.

Excess Alcohol

One may make the case that drinking alcohol in moderation does, in fact, have some positive health effects. This indicates that having a few drinks every once in a while isn't really going to hurt you all that much. On the other hand, consuming much more wine than is typical might lead to major health issues, including irritation. A disease known as irritable bowel syndrome may develop in those who have a problem with excessive drinking. This illness is characterized by the propensity of the body to store bacterial toxins. This illness has the potential to cause harm to several organs as well as extensive inflammation.

Artificial Trans Fats

Artificial Trans fats are without a doubt the unhealthiest fats that can be found anywhere on the earth. These are meals that include components that have been partially hydrogenated. This indicates that hydrogen is included in the production of unsaturated lipids. The majority of unsaturated fats exist in a liquid state. The addition of hydrogen causes them to become much more solid, which in turn increases their stability. Additionally, the quantity of HDL cholesterol in the body is decreased when artificial Tran's fats are consumed. Studies have shown that these substances also damage the sideothelial cells that line our arteries, which raises the probability that we may develop heart disease. Some varieties of pastries, cookies, and pre-packaged cakes, as well as margarine, vegetable shortening, French fries, oven popcorn, and other kinds of fast food, are typically prepared with artificial Tran's fats. Other foods that are typically prepared with artificial Trans fatty acids include oven popcorn, French fries, and other kinds of fast food.

Refined Carbs

It's not true that all carbohydrates are the same. There are some that are enjoyable to consume, and there are others that might be beneficial to have in your diet. To clarify, I'm talking to refined carbs when I say that the ones that are great to have but aren't really required. Take note that not all forms of carbohydrates pose a health risk. You have to understand that people have been eating carbohydrates ever since prehistoric times. It is a truth that our predecessors consumed unprocessed carbohydrates, which meant that their diets had a significant amount of fiber, which is beneficial to the body. On the other hand, during the process of refining, the fiber and all of the other important nutrients are removed.

The refined carbs are all that are still available to us. According to the study, even though they have a much longer shelf life, they may cause a significant amount of inflammation in the body. Keep in mind that fiber helps regulate blood sugar levels and that it generally makes you feel fuller for longer. When you have recently had a diet that was rich in fiber, you will not have a need for more food for this reason. Additionally, fiber nourishes the beneficial bacteria that are already present in your digestive tract, which contributes to the preservation of your general health.

Processed Meat

Beef jerky, ham, smoked meat, sausages, and bacon are all examples of processed cuts of meat. They have a wonderful flavor, and as a result, many people made them regulars at the dinner table. However, research suggests that consuming these foods may raise the risk of a number of other ailments, including stomach cancer, colon cancer, heart disease, and diabetes. Intake of processed meat is linked to the development of colon cancer more often than any other disease. Researchers believe that this could be because these meats have a high concentration of extended glycation side, also known as AGEs. AGEs are produced when high heat is applied to meat after it has been mixed with other components and then subjected to the mixture. Research backs up the theory that AGEs are to blame for inflammation throughout the body. Take into consideration the fact that the growth of colon cancer is influenced by a wide variety of variables. However, studies suggest that the intake of meat and the irritation that comes along with it is probably the single most important cause in the development of the disease.

CHAPTER 2: Anti-inflammatory Breakfast Recipes

2.1 Chia Seed and Milk Pudding

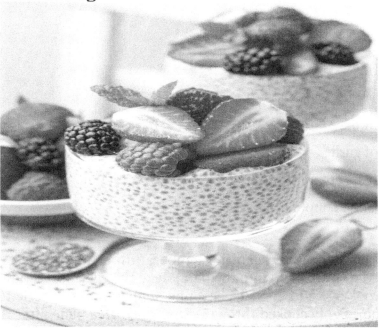

Preparation time: five Mins **Cooking time:** zero Mins **Serving:** 6 Persons

Ingredients

- one cup mixed berries (fresh, for garnishing)
- 4 cups coconut milk (full-fat)
- 3/4 cup coconut yogurt (for topping)
- quarter cup coconut chips (toasted for garnishing)
- half tsp cinnamon (ground)
- half cup chia seeds
- three tbsps honey
- one tsp vanilla extract
- one tsp turmeric (ground)
- half tsp ginger (ground)

Instructions

Mix the ginger, turmeric, and cinnamon in a mixing container along with the honey, vanilla essence, and coconut milk. Mix them well and continue to do so till the mixture takes on a yellowish hue. Include the chia seeds to the mixture and stir them around. Mix them thoroughly. For around five mins, you should refrain from stirring the mixture. After the first 5 mins have passed, give the mixture another stir. Cover the components together. Place it in the refrigerator, where it will stay for at least 6 hrs, preferably overnight. The pudding-like consistency will be achieved as a result of the chia seeds expanding and becoming plumper. Distribute the pudding among the four glasses. Put some coconut yogurt, coconut chips, and a combination of berries on top of each glass of pudding. Serve.

Nutrition Calories: 200 Kcal, Proteins: 12g, Fat: 8g, Carbohydrates: 21g

2.2 Scrambled Eggs with Turmeric
Preparation time: 6 Mins **Cooking time:** zero Mins **Serving:** 1 Person

Ingredients

- two radishes (grated)
- two kale leaves (shredded)
- 2 eggs (pastured)
- one tbsp turmeric
- two tbsps coconut oil
- one small clove of garlic (crushed)
- clover and radish sprouts (for topping)
- 1 tweak of of cayenne pepper

Instructions

Put some coconut oil in a pan and keep the temperature at moderate. Cook the garlic in the skillet. The eggs should be broken up into the pan. Make the eggs into scrambled form by stirring them while they are cooking. Add the kale, cayenne pepper, and turmeric to the scrambled eggs just before they are thoroughly cooked through. Stir. Place on a plate after the transfer. Radishes that have been grated and sprouts should be used as a topping. Serve.

Nutrition Calories: 401 Kcal, Proteins: 25g, Fat: 19g, Carbohydrates: 31g

---

2.3 Protein-Rich Turmeric Donuts
Preparation time: 5 Mins **Cooking time:** ten Mins **Serving:** one Person

Ingredients

- one and half cups cashews (raw)
- 7 Medjool dates (pitted)
- quarter cup coconut (shredded)
- one tbsp vanilla protein powder
- quarter cup dark chocolate (for topping)
- two tsps maple syrup
- quarter tsp vanilla essence
- one tsp turmeric powder

Instructions

Put all of the components, with the exception of the dark chocolate, into a mixing bowl and pulse till smooth. Mix on the highest speed till the mixture forms a dough that is silky smooth and sticky. Form the dough into a total of eight balls. Donuts should be made by pressing each ball tightly into a mold. Wrap the mold with a cover. Donuts will need to be chilled in the refrigerator for around half an hour. Put one cup of water into a pot and set it to cook over moderate heat. Start the water boiling in a pot. Put the dark chocolate in a smaller pot and start heating it up. Put the smaller pan on the upper edge of the bigger one that contains the water that is boiling. Chocolate should be stirred till it is thoroughly melted. Remove the doughnuts from the freezer and place them on a plate. Use the melted chocolate to create a glaze for the doughnuts. Serve.

Nutrition Calories: 323 Kcal, Proteins: 29g, Fat: 17g, Carbohydrates: 35g

2.4 Cranberry and Sweet Potato Bars
Preparation time: 6 Mins **Cooking time:** 10 Mins **Serving:** one Person

Ingredients

- one cup almond meal
- one and a half cups sweet potato purée
- one cup cranberries (fresh)
- one-third cup coconut flour
- quarter cup water
- two eggs
- two tbsps coconut oil (melted)
- 2 tbsps maple syrup
- one and a half tsp baking soda

Instructions

Turn the oven on to 350 °F and prepare the oven. Put the maple syrup, sweet potato puree, water, melted coconut oil, and eggs in a big container and mix well. Mix them together well. Sift the almond meal, coconut flour, and baking soda together in a distinct mixing container. Mix the components well. Mix the two dry components and include them to the liquid. Make sure the batter is well mixed. Prepare a 9-inch square baking dish by greasing it. Wrap parchment paper around the inside as well. The batter should be spread out on the prepared pan. Apply a thin layer of batter to the pan and spread it out evenly with a damp spoon. Put one berry at a time on top of a batter and press down gently. Put it in the oven and bake for 35 mins, checking it halfway through. When it's totally cold, cut it into 16 pieces.

Nutrition Calories: 130 Kcal, Proteins: 10g, Fat: 5g, Carbohydrates: 11g

---

2.5 Nutty Choco-Nana Pancakes
Preparation time: two Mins **Cooking time:** zero Mins **Serving:** two Persons

Ingredients

Pancakes:

- two eggs (big)
- 2 bananas (ripe)
- 2 tbsps creamy almond butter
- one-eighth tsp salt
- two tbsps cacao powder (raw)
- Coconut oil (for greasing)
- one tsp pure vanilla extract

Sauce:

- quarter cup coconut oil
- 4 tbsps cacao powder (raw)

Instructions

Pancakes: Get a pan ready on low heat. Grease the pan with one tbsp of coconut oil. Place everything you need to make pancakes into a mixing bowl. Mix all of the components together and pulse them on high till the batter is thoroughly smooth. To create one pancake, pour approximately a quarter cup of the mixture onto the hot skillet. Flip each pancake after 5 mins of cooking. Turn the pancake over very gently. For a further 2 mins, flip the meat. Repeat this process till no more batter is available. Sauce may be served alongside or on the pancakes.

Sauce: Warm the coconut oil in a pan over moderate heat. Add the cacao powder to the oil and stir till mixed. Get out of the sun. Leave aside.

Nutrition Calories: 621 Kcal, Proteins: 22.4g, Fat: 32g, Carbohydrates: 66g

2.6 Blueberry Avocado Chocolate Muffins
Preparation time: 15 Mins **Cooking time:** zero Mins **Serving:** two Persons

Ingredients

- half cup almond milk (unsweetened)
- one cup almond flour
- one-third cup coconut sugar
- quarter cup cacao powder + one tbsp (raw)
- quarter cup blueberries (fresh)
- two big eggs (room temp.)
- one small avocado (ripe)
- quarter tsp salt
- two tbsps coconut flour
- two tsps baking powder
- two tbsps dark chocolate chips

Instructions

Bake at 375 degrees Fahrenheit, which requires warming up the oven. Put paper muffin cups in a muffin tray. Put the eggs, salt, avocados, sugar, and 1 tbsp of the cacao powder in a mixer and mix till smooth. The texture should resemble smooth pudding after being mixed on high. Put everything in a big basin and stir it up. Sift the cocoa powder, baking soda, almond flour, and coconut flour into a big mixing basin. Mix the components well. Mix the avocado and almond milk and stir to mix. In a separate container, whisk together the flour and salt, then add it to the avocado combination and fold till everything is incorporated. Don't beat the mixture to death. Mix in the blueberries and chocolate chips. Spoon the mixture equally into the 9 prepared muffin cups. Put in the oven and cook for approximately 18 mins. Do not eat the muffins too warm.

Nutrition Calories: 130 Kcal, Proteins: 10.4g, Fat: 5g, Carbohydrates: 11g

2.7 Tropical Smoothie Container
Preparation time: 15 Mins **Cooking time:** zero Mins **Serving:** two Persons

Ingredients

- one cup orange juice
- one cup pineapple (frozen)
- 1 cup mango (frozen)
- half banana

- 1 spoonful of chia
- one-eighth tsp turmeric

Toppings:
- Kiwis (sliced)
- Coconut flakes
- Almonds (sliced)
- Strawberries (sliced)

Instructions

Place everything into a mixer and mix till smooth. Put them in a mixer and whirl them around till they form a smooth cream. If the mixture is excessively thick, a few drops of oranges at a time can do the trick. Split the smoothie in half and serve it in separate containers. Mix the components together and serve in individual containers. Serve.

Nutrition Calories: 230 Kcal, Proteins: 11.4g, Fat: 5g, Carbohydrates: 35g

2.8 Smoked Salmon in Scrambled Eggs
Preparation time: 10 Mins **Cooking time:** 0 Mins **Serving:** 1 Person

Ingredients

- 4 eggs
- four slices of smoked salmon (sliced)
- 3 stems of fresh chives (finely sliced)
- tweak of sea salt
- two tbsps coconut milk
- Pinch of black pepper (freshly ground)
- Cooking fat

Instructions

Coconut milk, chives, and eggs should all be mixd in a big container. Mix them with a whisk. Place salt and pepper on it. Beat the eggs in enough grease in a pan over moderate flame. The eggs should be poured into the pan. Scramble the eggs by stirring them. Scramble the eggs and add the fish. Add additional 2 mins to the cooking time. Serve.

Nutrition Calories: 205 Kcal, Proteins: 18.4g, Fat: 0.5g, Carbohydrates: 2.3g

2.9 Spinach and Potatoes with Smoked Salmon
Preparation time: ten Mins **Cooking time:** 0 Mins **Serving:** 1 Person

Ingredients

- two russet potatoes (skinned and diced)
- 4 eggs
- half onion (sliced)
- two cups baby spinach (fresh)
- 8 oz. smoked salmon (sliced)
- half cup mushrooms (sliced)

- two tbsps olive oil
- one garlic clove (crushed)
- two tbsps ghee
- half tsp garlic powder
- half tsp onion powder
- quarter tsp paprika
- Black pepper
- Sea salt

Instructions

Turn the oven temp. up to 425 degrees F. To prepare a baking dish, line it with parchment paper. Arrange the potatoes on the prepared baking sheet. Drizzle paprika, olive oil, onion powder, and garlic powder over the potatoes. Put pepper on it. Russet potatoes need thirty mins in the oven. At the halfway point, give the potatoes a flip. Put some water in a saucepan and set it over high heat. Let the water boil. Prepare a pot of boiling water for the eggs. Remove the heat source. Leave the eggs in the heated water for Seven mins. Remove the eggs from the cooker. The eggs should be rinsed under running water. Prepare the eggs by removing the shells. Place the ghee in a pot and melt it over moderate heat. In a skillet, heat the oil and sauté the garlic and onion for a few seconds. Place the mushrooms inside. Put salt and pepper on it. Add another 5 mins to the cooking time. Prepare the spinach and add it. Let them cook for 2 mins or till they are crumpled. Cut the brown potatoes into quarters and serve them evenly. Pile smoked salmon on top of the eggs and spinach combination, and serve. Serve.

Nutrition Calories: 205 Kcal, Proteins: 6g, Fat: 2.1g, Carbohydrates: 2.3g

2.10 Eggs in a Mushroom and Bacon

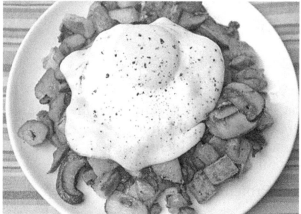

Preparation time: ten Mins **Cooking time:** zero Mins **Serving:** 4 Persons

Ingredients

- 4 Portobello mushroom caps
- 4 pasture-raised eggs (big)
- 2 strips thick-cut and pasture-raised bacon (cooked and sliced)
- one cup arugula
- 1 moderate tomato (sliced)
- Pepper

- Salt

Instructions

Set the oven temperature to 350 degrees F. So, have a baking sheet ready. Put parchment paper in it. Use a spoon to remove the heads from the mushrooms. Throw the gills away. Place the mushroom caps in a single layer on the prepared baking sheet. Put some arugula and diced tomatoes in each mushroom cap and serve. Put an egg over mushroom stems very carefully. Put the mushrooms in the center of the oven and bake for twenty mins. Put some bacon, salt, and pepper, on top of each mushroom. Serve.

Nutrition Calories: 124 Kcal, Proteins: 8g, Fat: 8.4g, Carbohydrates: 4.3g

2.11 Bacon Avocado Burger
Preparation time: ten Mins **Cooking time:** zero Mins **Serving:** 1 Person

Ingredients

- one ripe avocado
- 2 bacon rashers
- 1 red onion (sliced)
- 1 lettuce leaf
- 1 egg
- Sea salt
- 1 tomato (sliced)
- Sesame seeds (for garnishing)
- 1 tbsp Paleo mayonnaise

Instructions

Carefully place the bacon in the pan. To warm up the stove, set the temp. to moderate. Brown the bacon. Whenever the bacon rashers flare, flip them with a fork. Keep frying till they reach the desired crispiness. Don't eat any more of that deliciously crispy bacon right now. Break the egg into the same pan you used to cook the bacon. Make a fried egg in bacon grease. It is ideal for the egg white to be firm but the yolk to be soft. Put the finished egg to one side. You should halve the avocado lengthwise. Dig that hole out! Remove the meat by spooning it out of the skin. Spread the mayonnaise into the empty space left by the avocado. Spread the avocado on a plate, and then layer on the bacon, egg, tomato, and onion. Drizzle some salt over it. Complete the layer by slicing the rest of the avocado in half and spreading it on top. Drizzle some sesame seeds on top. Serve.

Nutrition Calories: 440 Kcal, Proteins: 37g, Fat: 49g, Carbohydrates: 51g

2.12 Spinach Fry Up & Tomato Mushroom
Preparation time: ten Mins **Cooking time:** 5 Mins **Serving:** two Persons

Ingredients

- 3 big handfuls of English spinach leaves (torn)
- 6 button mushrooms (sliced)
- A handful of cherry tomatoes (sliced in halves)
- 1 garlic clove (finely diced)
- Drizzle of lemon juice

- half red onion (sliced)
- two tbsps olive oil
- half tsp lemon zest (grated)
- one tsp ghee
- half tsp sea salt
- Pinch of black pepper (ground)
- Pinch of nutmeg

Instructions

Put the olive oil and ghee in a pan and heat them over moderate flame. The mushrooms and onions should be cooked in a sautéing pan till tender. Tomatoes, lemon, and garlic rind should be mixd and stirred together. Add some salt, pepper, and nutmeg for flavor. Add additional 2 mins to the cooking time. Make the crushed tomato sauce by mashing tomatoes with a spoon. Include the spinach leaves and mix. Wilt them in the cooking process. Put some lime juice on it. Serve.

Nutrition Calories: 61.5 Kcal, Proteins: 3.3g, Fat: 2.5g, Carbohydrates: 6.6g

2.13 Chocolate Milkshake

Preparation time: 12 Mins **Cooking time:** 5 Mins **Serving:** two Persons

Ingredients

- 4 ice cubes
- two big organic bananas (frozen)
- half tsp vanilla extract
- one cup coconut milk
- two tbsps cashew butter
- one tbsp cacao powder (raw)

Instructions

Place the coconut cream and bananas in a mixer or mixing bowl and mix till smooth. Double or triple pulse. Stir in the cocoa powder, nut butter, and flavoring. Repeat the process two or three times. Fill it up with ice. Put everything in a mixer and whir it up till it's thoroughly mixd. The consistency of the milkshake may be adjusted as required by adding additional ice cubes or coconut milk. Fill a glass with it. Serve.

Nutrition Calories: 371 Kcal, Proteins: 8.2g, Fat: 17g, Carbohydrates: 51g

2.14 Almond Sweet Cherry Chia Pudding

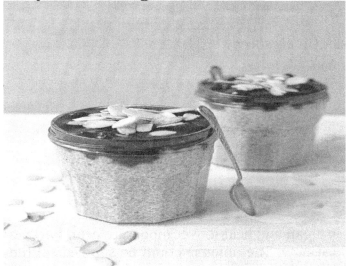

Preparation time: 15 Mins **Cooking time:** Mins **Serving:** 2 Persons

Ingredients

- 2 cups whole sweet cherries (pitted)
- 3/4 cup chia seeds
- half cup hemp seeds
- quarter cup maple syrup
- 13.5 oz. can coconut milk
- 1 tsp vanilla extract
- 1 tsp almond extract
- one-eighth tsp sea salt

Topping:

1. four servings of cherry

Instructions

The cherries, vanilla extract, coconut milk, almond extract, salt, and maple syrup should be mixed together. They should be mixed till they are thoroughly smooth. Add the chia seeds and hemp seeds. Put everything in the mixer and mix on a low speed to mix. Divide it across 4 glasses. Allow the pudding to chill in the refrigerator for a minimum of an hour. Cherry, each pudding to finish it off. Serve.

Nutrition Calories: 242 Kcal, Proteins: 7g, Fat: 11g, Carbohydrates: 33g

2.15 Shakshuka

Preparation time: 10 Mins **Cooking time:** Mins **Serving:** 6 Persons

Ingredients

- 6 eggs (big)
- 4 cups tomatoes (diced)
- half onion (sliced)
- Sea salt
- 1 clove of garlic (crushed)

- 1 red bell pepper (sliced and seeded)
- 2 tbsps tomato paste
- half tbsp fresh parsley (finely sliced)
- 1 tbsp cooking fat
- 1 tsp paprika
- Pinch of cayenne pepper
- 1 tsp chili powder
- Black pepper

Instructions

Place the lard for frying in a pan and heat it over moderate heat. For two mins, sauté the onions. The garlic should be added now. The onions should be sautéed till they are soft. Add the bell pepper and mix well. Wait till the chills are tsideer before serving. Tomatoes, chili powder, paprika, cayenne pepper, and tomato paste should be stirred in. Add salt and pepper as required. Temper the heat a little. The components should be heated for several mins at a low simmer. The eggs should be broken over the mixture while it is still boiling. Spread the eggs out equally. Keep the skillet covered. Keep it at a heat till the eggs are done. Top with sliced parsley. Serve.

Nutrition Calories: 298 Kcal, Proteins: 17g, Fat: 19g, Carbohydrates: 16g

2.16 Anti-Inflammatory Salad
Preparation time: 12 Mins **Cooking time:** Mins **Serving:** 4 Persons

Ingredients

Dressing:
- 1 clove of garlic (grated)
- one-third cup extra virgin olive oil
- 2 tbsps apple cider vinegar
- 1 tbsp lemon juice
- 1 tsp turmeric
- 1 tsp fresh ginger (grated)
- half tsp sea salt
- quarter tsp black pepper (freshly ground)

Salad:
- 16 oz. beets (cooked, skinned, and sliced)
- 2 12-ounce bags of Trader Joe's Sweet Kale Salad Mix
- 1 half cup blueberries (fresh)

Instructions

Put the dressing components in a mixer and mix till smooth. The salad components should be split between six containers. Dress with a drizzle. Serve.

Nutrition Calories: 20 Kcal, Proteins: 17g, Fat: 19g, Carbohydrates: 16g

2.17 Amaranth Porridge with Pears
Preparation time: 12 Mins **Cooking time:** 5 Mins **Serving:** 4 Persons

Ingredients

Pears:

- 1 tsp maple syrup
- 1 pear (big and diced)
- half tsp cinnamon (ground)
- quarter tsp ginger (ground)
- one-eighth tsp nutmeg (ground)
- one-eighth tsp clove (ground)

Porridge:

- half cup amaranth (uncooked, drained, and rinsed)
- half cup water
- 1 cup 2% milk
- quarter tsp salt

Topping:

- 1 cup 0% Greek yogurt (plain)
- 2 tbsps pecan pieces
- 1 tsp maple syrup (pure)

Instructions

Turn the oven temperature up to 400 degrees F. Prepare parchment paper on a baking pan. Put all of the porridge components into a saucepan and cook them over moderate. Get the water boiling? Turn down the stove. Allow the porridge to cook for a quarter of an hour. Putting aside. The pecan bits should be spread out on the prepared baking sheet. Spread maple syrup all over them. On the same baking sheet covered with pecan bits, place the diced pears. Pour some maple syrup over the pears. Bake them in the oven for fifteen mins. Stir the fruits into the cereal. Keep some pears for sprinkling. Two cups of porridge, please. Put some yogurt in each of the dishes. Porridge should be served in containers. Add the rest of the pears and pecans to the top of each serving of porridge. Serve.

Nutrition Calories: 500 Kcal, Proteins: 78g, Fat: 1.5g, Carbohydrates: 8g

2.18 Sweet Potato Breakfast Container
Preparation time: 15 Mins **Cooking time:** 5 Mins **Serving:** 3 Persons

Ingredients

- 1 small banana (sliced)
- 1 small sweet potato (pre-baked)
- quarter cup raspberries
- 1 serving protein powder
- quarter cup blueberries

Toppings:

- Favorite nuts
- Chia seeds
- Cacao nibs
- Hemp hearts

Instructions

Purée the sweet potato in a container. Add the protein powder and mix well. Mix. Arrange the bananas, raspberries, and blueberries on top. Drizzle on the condiments after. Serve.

Nutrition Calories: 210 Kcal, Proteins: 3.8g, Fat: 1.3g, Carbohydrates: 48g

2.19 Apple Turkey Hash
Preparation time: 20 Mins **Cooking time:** 0 Mins **Serving:** 4 Persons

Ingredients
Hash:

- 2 cups spinach
- 2 cups frozen butternut squash (cubed)
- half cup carrots (shredded)
- 1 big apple (skinned, cored, and sliced)
- 1 onion
- 1 big zucchini
- 1 tsp cinnamon
- 1 tbsp coconut oil
- half tsp thyme (dried)
- half tsp garlic powder
- half tsp turmeric
- 3/4 tsp powdered ginger
- Sea salt

Meat:

- half tsp thyme (dried)
- 1 pound ground turkey
- 1 tbsp coconut oil
- half tsp cinnamon
- Sea salt

Instructions

Put the coconut oil in a pan and heat it over moderate heat. When the turkey is done, add it to the pan and stir it in. Add some salt, pepper, cinnamon, and thyme as required. Putting aside. Toss the coconut oil into the same pan and heat it over moderate heat. Lighten the onions by sautéing them. Mix in the apples, butternut squash, carrots, and zucchini. Make sure they're cooked all the way through so they're nice and tender. Mix in the spinach. If you want it wilted, cook it longer. Add the crushed turkey and mix it with the other components. Serve.

Nutrition Calories: 325 Kcal, Proteins: 28g, Fat: 19g, Carbohydrates: 20g

2.20 Oats with Almonds and Blueberries
Preparation time: 15 Mins **Cooking time:** 0 Mins **Serving:** 4 Persons

Ingredients

Oats:

- 3/4 cup old-fashioned oats
- 3/4 cup almond milk
- 1 tbsp maple syrup

Toppings:

- quarter cup blueberries
- one-third cup yogurt
- 3 tbsps almonds (sliced)

Instructions

Scoop the oats into a canning jar (1-pint). Mix the almond milk and maple syrup well in a container. Mix the milk and honey into the oats. Lock the lid on the jar. Reserve in the refrigerator for at least eight hrs, preferably overnight. Fill it with condiments. Serve.

Nutrition Calories: 230 Kcal, Proteins: 8g, Fat: 5g, Carbohydrates: 40g

2.21 Chia Energy Bars with Chocolate
Preparation time: 12 Mins **Cooking time:** 0 Mins **Serving:** 4 Persons

Ingredients

- 1 cup walnut pieces (raw)
- 1 half cups pitted dates (packed)
- one-third cup cacao powder (raw)
- half cup whole chia seeds
- half cup coconut shavings
- 1 tsp pure vanilla extract
- half cup dark chocolate (sliced)
- quarter tsp sea salt (unrefined)
- half cup oats

Instructions

Place the dates into the food processor. Prepare a thick paste by processing. Place it in a basin for mixing. Drop the walnuts in there. Ensure an in-depth mixing. Add the last of the components. Knead it till it creates a ball of dough. Obtain a square dish for baking. Prepare the dish by lining it with baking parchment. Place the mixture on the prepared baking sheet. Evenly disperse the dough, and then push it down firmly into the dish. Freeze for at least a few hrs and up to a full day. Cube into 14 pieces. Serve.

Nutrition Calories: 234 Kcal, Proteins: 4.5g, Fat: 12g, Carbohydrates: 28g

2.22 Baked Rice Porridge with Maple and Fruit
Preparation time: 15 Mins **Cooking time:** 0 Mins **Serving:** 5 Persons

Ingredients

- 2 tbsps pure maple syrup
- half cup brown rice
- half tsp pure vanilla extract
- Pinch of cinnamon
- Sliced fruits (berries, plums, pears, or cherries)
- Pinch of salt

Instructions

Turn the oven temperature up to 400 degrees F. Brown rice and a glass of water should be cooked together in a saucepan over moderate heat. Get the water boiling. Mix with some vanilla bean paste and cinnamon. Cover. Turn down the stove. Allow the rice to boil till it is done. Toss the rice every once in a while. Have two containers that can go from fridge to oven ready. Assign each container the same amount of rice. Drizzle some maple syrup and sliced fruits over the rice. Put some salt on it. Put in the oven and set the timer for 15 mins. Serve.

Nutrition Calories: 228 Kcal, Proteins: 3.5g, Fat: 1.5g, Carbohydrates: 50g

2.23 Banana Chia Pudding

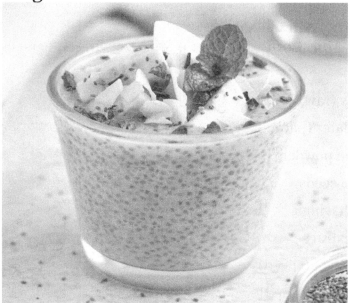

Preparation time: 20 Mins **Cooking time:** 0 Mins **Serving:** 5 Persons

Ingredients

- half cup chia seeds
- 2 cups almond milk (unsweetened)
- 1 big banana (very ripe)
- half tsp pure vanilla extract
- 2 tbsp maple syrup
- 1 tbsp cacao powder

Mix-ins:

- 2 tbsps chocolate chips
- 2 tbsps cacao nibs
- 1 big banana (sliced)

Instructions

Put the banana and chia seeds in a big container and stir them together. Mix the components by mashing them well. Mix the milk and vanilla essence and add to the pan. Mix well to eliminate any lumps. Get two sealed containers ready. To divide the chia seeds in half, divide the mixture between two containers. Cover. The rest of the portion of the hemp seeds combination should be mixd with maple syrup and cacao powder. Make sure everything is well mixed. Transfer the compound to the secondary container. Cover. These containers should be refrigerated for at least a few hrs, preferably overnight. Divide the chia pudding and the toppings into 3 glasses and layer. Serve.

Nutrition Calories: 260 Kcal, Proteins: 6g, Fat: 5g, Carbohydrates: 60g

2.24 Baked Eggs with Herbs

Preparation time: 15 Mins **Cooking time:** 10 Mins **Serving:** 5 Persons

Ingredients

2. A tbsp of milk
3. A sprinkling of dried herbs like thyme, oregano, parsley, garlic powder, and dill
4. A tsp of melted butter,
5. Two eggs

Instructions

Turn the oven's broiler on to a low level and warm up it. Put the butter and milk in a moderate baking dish. Combo together successfully. Spread the butter-milk combo all over the baking dish. Separate the eggs and place them in the dish. Top with a sprinkling of herbs and garlic. Put it in the oven for a couple of mins so the eggs can bake.

Nutrition Calories: 341 Kcal, Proteins: 20g, Fat: 27g, Carbohydrates: 3g

2.25 Banana Bread Pecan Overnight Oats

Preparation time: 20 Mins **Cooking time:** 0 Mins **Serving:** 5 Persons

Ingredients

- 1 cup old-fashioned rolled oats
- 1 half cups milk
- quarter cup Greek yogurt (plain)
- 2 tbsps honey
- 2 bananas (very ripe, mashed)
- 2 tbsps coconut flakes
- quarter tsp sea salt (flaked)
- 1 tbsp chia seeds
- 2 tsps vanilla extract

Topping:

- Banana slices

- Roasted pecans
- Honey
- Pomegranate seeds
- Fig halves

Instructions

To prepare, mix the oats, coconut flakes, bananas, milk, yogurt, honey, chia seeds, vanilla, and sea salt essence in a big mixing dish. Mix together well. Place the oat mixture into two containers and divide it in half. Cover. The recommended minimum time in the fridge is 6 hrs, but overnight is best. Toss the components together and stir. Add the toppings to each plate of oats and serve. Serve.

Nutrition Calories: 370 Kcal, Proteins: 16g, Fat: 8g, Carbohydrates: 58g

2.26 Cinnamon Granola with Fruits

Preparation time: 15 Mins **Cooking time:** 0 Mins **Serving:** 5 Persons

Ingredients

- quarter cup walnuts (sliced)
- 2 cups old-fashioned rolled oats
- quarter cup shredded coconut (unsweetened)
- quarter cup dried apricots (sliced)
- quarter cup honey
- quarter cup raisins
- 4 tbsps unsalted butter (melted)
- quarter tsp ground cloves
- quarter cup dried cranberries
- 2 tbsps pumpkin seeds
- quarter tsp ground nutmeg
- half tsp ground cinnamon

Instructions

Turn the oven temperature up to three hundred degrees F. To prepare a baking sheet, line it with parchment paper. Mix the oats, pumpkin seeds, spices, coconuts, walnuts, and salt in a big mixing basin. Don't bother with it right now. Throw the honey and butter into a separate container. Combo together successfully. Add the liquid to the oats and stir. Combo together successfully. Put the oat mix on the prepared baking sheet. The spread was uniform. Put in the oven and bake for 20-25 mins. Let it cool down a little. Prepare the granola by breaking it up. Mix the granola pieces and dried fruit. Put away in a container with a tight lid.

Nutrition Calories: 120 Kcal, Proteins: 2g, Fat: 4.5g, Carbohydrates: 18g

2.27 Yogurt Parfait with Chia Seeds and Raspberries

Preparation time: 20 Mins **Cooking time:** 0 Mins **Serving:** 5 Persons

Ingredients

- 16 oz. yogurt (plain, divided into 4 portions)

- half cup raspberries (fresh)
- 2 tbsps chia seeds
- 1 tsp maple syrup
- Pinch of cinnamon

Topping:

- Nectarines (sliced)
- Strawberries (sliced)
- Blackberries (sliced)

Instructions

Place the raspberries in a big basin. Mix them and mash them till they resemble jam. Mix with some cinnamon and honey with some chia seeds. Put everything in a mixer and blitz it till it's a uniform consistency. Divide into halves and set aside. Put two in the glass. Spread some yogurt on the bottom of each cup. The raspberry filling comes next. The last layer consists of any leftover yogurt. Incorporate the condiments. Serve.

Nutrition Calories: 252 Kcal, Proteins: 13g, Fat: 12g, Carbohydrates: 25g

2.28 Avocado Toast with Egg

Preparation time: 15 Mins **Cooking time:** 10 Mins **Serving:** 4 Persons

Ingredients

- 1 slice of gluten-free bread (toasted)
- 1 half tsp ghee
- 1 egg (scrambled)
- Red pepper flakes
- half avocado (sliced)
- A handful of spinach leaves

Instructions

Apply some ghee to the hot toast. Layer the toast with avocado slices. Spinach leaves are a great garnish. The scrambled egg should be served on top. Add some crushed red pepper for heat. Serve.

Nutrition Calories: 260 Kcal, Proteins: 12g, Fat: 16g, Carbohydrates: 20g

2.29 Winter Morning Breakfast Container

Preparation time: 15 Mins **Cooking time:** 0 Mins **Serving:** 4 Persons

Ingredients

- 1 cup of quinoa
- 2 half cups coconut water
- 2 whole cloves
- 1-star anise pod
- 1 cinnamon stick

Fresh Fruits:

- Blackberries
- Apples
- Cranberries
- Persimmons
- Pears

Instructions

Put the coconut water, quinoa, and seasonings into a pot and cook it over moderate heat. Simmer them till they reach a rolling boil. Put the lid on it. Turn down the stove. The recommended cooking time is 25 mins. Split the quinoa in half and place it in separate dishes. Do not use entire spices. Put some fruit on top of each dish. Serve.

Nutrition Calories: 257 Kcal, Proteins: 12g, Fat: 8g, Carbohydrates: 40g

2.30 Broccoli and Quinoa Breakfast Patties

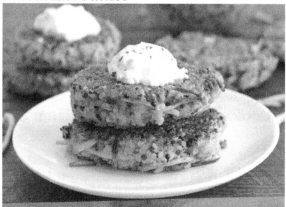

Preparation time: 5 Mins **Cooking time:** 6 Mins **Serving:** 3 Persons

Ingredients

- half cup shredded broccoli florets
- 1 cup cooked quinoa, cooked
- half cup shredded carrots
- 2 tsp parsley
- 2 cloves of garlic, crushed
- 1 half tsp onion powder
- one-third tsp salt
- 1 half tsp garlic powder
- quarter tsp black pepper
- 2 tbsp coconut oil
- half cup bread crumbs, gluten-free
- 2 flax eggs

Instructions

To make the patties, put all of the components (excluding the oil) in a big container and whisk till smooth. To make the patties, heat the oil in a skillet over moderate heat, add the patties once the oil is heated (about 3 mins on each side), and then remove them from the fire. Prepare vegan sour creams to accompany the burgers.

Nutrition Calories: 190 Kcal, Proteins: 9g, Fat: 5g, Carbohydrates: 23g

2.31 Scrambled Tofu Breakfast Tacos

Preparation time: 5 Mins **Cooking time:** 10 Mins **Serving:** 4 Persons

Ingredients

1. half cup grape tomatoes, quartered
2. 12 oz. tofu, pressed, drained
3. 1 moderate red pepper, diced
4. 1 clove of garlic, crushed
5. 8 corn tortillas
6. 1 moderate avocado, sliced
7. quarter tsp ground turmeric
8. 1 tsp olive oil
9. quarter tsp salt
10. quarter tsp ground black pepper
11. quarter tsp cumin

Instructions

Put the oil in a skillet and heat it over a moderate flame; when the oil is heated, add the garlic and pepper and sauté for two mins. Crumble in some tofu, season it with salt, black pepper, and all the seasonings, and cook it for 5 mins while stirring occasionally. When ready, divide the tofu among the tortillas, then top with the tomato and avocado.

Nutrition Calories: 240 Kcal, Proteins: 12g, Fat: 8g, Carbohydrates: 26g

2.32 Potato Skillet Breakfast

Preparation time: 5 Mins **Cooking time:** 15 Mins **Serving:** 5 Persons

Ingredients

- 1 quarter pounds potatoes, diced
- 1 half cup cooked black beans
- 12 oz. spinach
- 2 small avocados, sliced, for topping
- 1 quarter pounds red potatoes, diced
- 1 moderate green bell pepper, diced
- 1 big white onion, diced
- 1 jalapeno, crushed
- 1 moderate red bell pepper, diced
- half tsp red chili powder
- 3 cloves of garlic, crushed
- quarter tsp salt
- 1 tbsp canola oil
- 1 tsp cumin

Instructions

A warmed up oven is ready in a short amount of time, so turn it on and set the temperature to 425 degrees F. Secondly, heat the oil in a skillet over moderate heat. When the oil is heated, add the potatoes and cook, often stirring, for 2 mins before seasoning with salt, chili powder, and cumin. Put the pan in the oven and bake the potatoes for twenty mins, tossing once halfway through till they are done. After 15 mins, add the rest of the onion, garlic, bell peppers, and jalapeño and continue roasting, turning once halfway through. Place skillet over moderate heat and cook for 5-10 mins, occasionally stirring, till potatoes are tender. Add beans and spinach and simmer for another 3 mins, occasionally stirring, till basil leaves have wilted. When finished, drizzle the pan with sliced cilantro and serve with avocado.

Nutrition Calories: 199 Kcal, Proteins: 4g, Fat: 7g, Carbohydrates: 32g

2.33 Peanut Butter and Banana Bread Granola

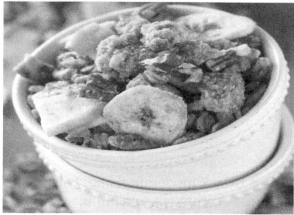

Preparation time: 10 Mins **Cooking time:** 32 Mins **Serving:** 6 Persons

Ingredients

1. half cup mashed banana
2. half cup Quinoa
3. 3 cup rolled oats, old-fashioned
4. 1 cup peanuts, salted
5. 1 cup banana chips, crushed
6. 1 tsp. salt
7. quarter cup brown sugar
8. 1 tsp. cinnamon
9. quarter cup honey
10. one-third cup peanut butter
11. 2 tsps. vanilla extract, unsweetened
12. 6 tbsps. unsalted butter

Instructions

Turn on the oven and prepare it for 325 degrees Fahrenheit. Prepare two lined baking trays ahead of time by lining them with parchment paper and setting them away. Stir together the oats, banana chips, quinoa, cinnamon, sugar, and salt in a container. Put the butter and nectar in a small pan and heat them over low flame, often stirring, for about 4 mins, or till the honey has melted. Then, take the pan off the heat and toss in the banana and vanilla till well mixed.

Finally, add this to the grain mixture and mix to mix. Cook the granola for 20-25 mins, till golden brown, dividing the mixture equally between two baking pans. Cool the granola thoroughly on the baking sheets set over wire racks before breaking it up and serving. As soon as possible, serve.

Nutrition Calories: 655 Kcal, Proteins: 18g, Fat: 36g, Carbohydrates: 70g

2.34 Chocolate Chip, Strawberry and Oat Waffles
Preparation time: 10 Mins **Cooking time:** 25 Mins **Serving:** 6 Persons

Ingredients

1. 6 tbsps chocolate chips, semi-sweet
2. quarter tsp salt
3. half cup sliced strawberries
4. 2 tsps baking powder

Wet Ingredients:

- one-third cup mashed bananas
- Powdered sugar as needed for topping

Dry Ingredients:

- quarter cup oats
- 2 tbsp maple syrup
- 2 tbsp coconut oil
- half tsp vanilla extract, unsweetened
- 1 half tbsp ground flaxseeds
- 1 half cup whole wheat pastry flour
- 2 half tbsp cocoa powder
- quarter cup applesauce, unsweetened
- 1 3/4 cup almond milk, unsweetened

Instructions

Put the dry components in a moderate container and whisk them together. Put the liquid components in a moderate container and mix till mixed. Add the dry components and whisk in four separate batches just till mixed. In the meanwhile, turn on the griddle and let it heat up to a high temperature while you let the batter sit out at ambient temperature for Five mins. Then, spoon in a sixth of the mixture and bake till the pancake is firm and golden. Keep making waffles in a similar fashion till all the batter is gone, then drizzle the finished waffles with sugar and top with cocoa powder and fruit.

Nutrition Calories: 261 Kcal, Proteins: 6g, Fat: 10g, Carbohydrates: 41g

2.35 Chickpea Flour Omelet
Preparation time: 5 Mins **Cooking time:** 12 Mins **Serving:** 1 Person

Ingredients

- Approximately one-half of a tsp of sliced chives
- quarter cup of chickpea flour
- half cup of sliced spinach

- quarter tsp. of garlic powder
- Exactly a Cup and a Tbsp of Water
- A tweak of of turmeric
- Black pepper, ground, one-eighth tsp
- half tsp of yeast extract
- The equivalent of half a tsp of baking powder
- half tsp. egg substitute for vegans

Instructions

Put everything, save from the spinach, in a container and whisk to incorporate. Set aside for 5 mins. Then, heat some oil in a skillet and set it over low heat. When the pan is heated, add the components and let them cook for three mins or till the edges are dry. Then place spinach over half of the omelet, fold over the other half, and cook for 2 mins more. The omelet should be slid onto a platter and served with ketchup.

Nutrition Calories: 151 Kcal, Proteins: 10g, Fat: 2g, Carbohydrates: 24g

CHAPTER 3: Anti-Inflammatory Lunch Recipes

3.1 Buddha Container with Avocado, Wild Rice, Kale, and Orange

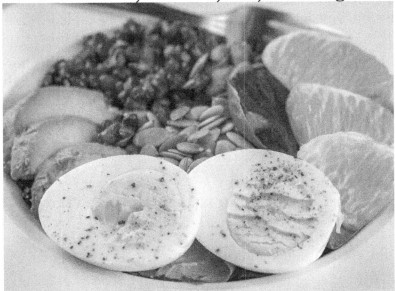

Preparation time: 15 Mins **Cooking time:** 12 Mins **Serving:** 4 Persons

Ingredients

Rice:

- 1 cup wild rice
- 3 cups vegetable broth
- 1 garlic clove (crushed)
- 2 tbsps extra-virgin olive oil
- 2 tbsps rice vinegar
- 1 tbsp fresh mint (sliced)
- Salt
- Freshly ground black pepper

Toppings:

- quarter cup pumpkin seeds
- quarter cup pomegranate seeds
- 1 bunch kale (roughly sliced)
- Salt
- 1 orange (segmented)
- 2 eggs (hard-boiled)
- half avocado (sliced)
- 2 tbsps olive oil
- 1 tbsp rice vinegar
- Freshly ground black pepper

Instructions

Rice: Put the broth, garlic, and rice in a saucepan and simmer it over moderate heat. Mix components by stirring. Get it boiling. Turn down the stove. Allow the rice to simmer for fifteen min or till cooked, and all liquid has been absorbed. Wait 10 mins before serving so the rice can cool down. Mint, olive oil, vinegar, salt, and pepper should be added. Mix thoroughly with the rice by tossing.

Toppings: Mix the kale, olive oil, and vinegar in a big container. Mix together by giving it a good toss. Divide the rice in half and put it in two separate dishes. Drizzle the kale mixture over the rice in each dish. Spread the rest of the condiments across the two serving dishes evenly. Add some salt and pepper for flavor. Serve.

Nutrition Calories: 1059 Kcal, Proteins: 65g, Fat: 38g, Carbohydrates: 108g

3.2 Avocado Chickpea Salad Sandwich

Preparation time: 12 Mins **Cooking time:** 15 Mins **Serving:** 6 Persons

Ingredients

- 1 15-ounce-can chickpea (drained and rinsed)
- 1 big avocado (ripe)
- Freshly ground pepper
- 2 tsps lime juice
- quarter cup cranberries (dried)
- 4 slices of whole grain bread
- Salt

Toppings:

- Arugula
- Red onion
- Spinach

Instructions

Put the chickpeas in a big basin and stir them around. Use a fork to mix them up. Prepare the avocado by placing it inside. Keep crushing it till it's mostly fine with some lumpy bits. Cranberries and fresh lemon juice should be added. Add some salt and pepper for flavor. Mix in a harmonious manner. The bread should be toasted. The chickpea mixture should be divided in half. Spread one serving onto a piece of toast. Apply your preferred toppings on the top. Add another piece of bread to finish the sandwich. Serve.

Nutrition Calories: 340 Kcal, Proteins: 15g, Fat: 12g, Carbohydrates: 46g

3.3 Spiced Lentil Soup

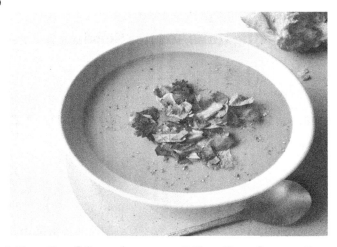

Preparation time: 20 Mins **Cooking time:** 20 Mins **Serving:** 4 Persons

Ingredients

- 3/4 cup red lentils (rinsed, uncooked, and drained)
- 3 half cups vegetable broth (low-sodium)
- 1 half tbsps extra-virgin olive oil
- 1 big onion (diced)
- 2 garlic cloves (crushed)
- Freshly ground black pepper
- 1 14-ounce-can coconut milk (full-fat)
- 1 5-ounce-package baby spinach
- 1 14-ounce-can diced tomatoes (with juice)
- 2 tsps turmeric (ground)
- 1 half tsps cumin (ground)
- 2 tsps fresh lime juice
- half tsp fine sea salt
- quarter tsp cardamom (ground)
- half tsp cinnamon
- Cayenne pepper

Instructions

Put the oil into a pan and heat it over moderate heat. To soften the onion, sauté it with garlic and salt. Cardamom, turmeric, cumin, and cinnamon should be added now. Mix components by stirring. Continue cooking for one minute. Mix in the red lentils, broth, cayenne pepper, black pepper, coconut milk, and salt. Mix well by stirring. Let the liquid reach a rolling boil. Turn down the stove. Allow the components to boil for twenty mins. Soft and airy le nails are ideal. Take it away from the stove. Do not forget the spinach! Mix components by stirring. Add some salt, pepper, and lime juice for seasoning. Serve.

Nutrition Calories: 331 Kcal, Proteins: 30g, Fat: 3.6g, Carbohydrates: 47.5g

3.4 Red Lentil Pasta with Tomato
Preparation time: 15 Mins **Cooking time:** 10 Mins **Serving:** 4 Persons

Ingredients

- quarter cup extra virgin olive oil
- half cup sun-dried tomatoes (oil-packed, drained, and sliced)
- 6 cloves garlic (crushed)
- 2 big handfuls of kale
- 1 sweet onion (sliced)
- 1 can (28 oz.) fire roasted tomatoes
- 1 tbsp oregano (dried)
- 1 box (8 oz.) of red lentil pasta
- 1 tbsp basil (dried)
- 2 tsps turmeric (ground)
- 1 tbsp apple cider vinegar
- Pepper
- Toasted pine nuts (for topping)
- Kosher salt

Instructions

Put the oil into a pan and heat it over moderate heat. The onion should be sautéed for 5 mins or till tsideer. Garlic, basil, oregano, turmeric, salt, and pepper should be stirred in. Continue cooking for one minute. Roasted tomatoes, please (juice included). Stir the tomatoes till they are crushed. Add the solar tomatoes and balsamic vinegar. Put the pot on low heat and simmer for fifteen min. Toss the greens in and mix it up. 5 additional mins of cooking time are required. The red lentil spaghetti should be prepared as directed on the box. Divide the spaghetti into 6 containers into equal amounts. Drizzle some pine nuts and tomato sauce on top of each container. Serve.

Nutrition Calories: 270 Kcal, Proteins: 8.5g, Fat: 4.5g, Carbohydrates: 49g

3.5 Tuna Mediterranean Salad
Preparation time: 15 Mins **Cooking time:** 05 Mins **Serving:** 4 Persons

Ingredients

- 1 14.5-ounce-can chickpea (drained and rinsed)
- 2 cans Albacore Tuna (drained)
- 1 cup red peppers (roasted and sliced)
- half cup pepperocini (diced)
- one-third cup parsley (finely sliced)
- quarter cup feta cheese
- 1 cucumber (sliced)
- half red onion (diced)

- 2 tsps capers
- Pinch of fine sea salt
- Sundried tomatoes (sliced)
- Olives
- Pinch of black pepper

Dressing:
- 2 tbsps olive oil
- Pinch black pepper
- 2 tbsps red wine vinegar
- 1 tsp lemon juice
- Pinch fine salt
- 1 tsp dried parsley
- 1 tsp dried oregano

Instructions

Put everything for the salad into a big mixing basin. Throw everything for the dressing into a separate dish. Stir the whisk vigorously. Coat the salad with the dressing. Throw everything together in a container and toss. Serve with half of an avocado.

Nutrition Calories: 230 Kcal, Proteins: 28g, Fat: 10g, Carbohydrates: 40g

3.6 Chicken and Greek Salad Wrap
Preparation time: 15 Mins **Cooking time:** 25 Mins **Serving:** 2 Persons

Ingredients
- 1 tbsp olive oil (divided)
- 2 chicken breasts (bone-in)
- half tsp dried oregano
- half tsp lemon pepper
- half tsp garlic powder

Salad:
- one-third cup feta cheese
- 4 cups romaine (sliced)
- one-third cup cherry tomatoes (sliced)
- quarter cup red onion
- red wine vinegar
- half cup cucumber slices (sliced)
- 4 tbsps hummus
- half tsp dried oregano
- 2 tbsps kalamata olives
- 2 gluten-free wraps

- olive oil
- 1 fresh lemon wedge (juiced)

Instructions

Salad: Put the romaine, cucumbers, tomatoes, onion, oregano, cheese, and olives in a container and toss. Use duality of the vinegar, one twist of the canola oil, and the juice of half a lemon to dress the salad. Mix by tossing.

Chicken: Bake at 375 degrees Fahrenheit, which requires warm uping the oven. Prepare a foil-lined baking sheet. Use a drizzle of olive oil, around half of the whole amount. The chicken should be placed on the prepared baking sheet. Add some salt, pepper, pepper flakes, garlic powder, oregano, and lemon pepper for flavor. Using the rest of the olive oil, drizzle the mixture. Bake at 400 degrees for 40 mins. Completely chill the chicken before serving. Cut into manageable chunks.

Wrap: Smear each wrap with 2 tbsps of hummus. Add the salad and chicken pieces in layers. Wrap. Serve.

Nutrition Calories: 230 Kcal, Proteins: 39g, Fat: 28g, Carbohydrates: 22g

3.7 Cauliflower and Chickpea Coconut Curry
Preparation time: 15 Mins **Cooking time:** 25 Mins **Serving:** 2 Persons

Ingredients

- 1 can (14 oz.) of coconut milk
- 1 can (28 oz.) of cooked chickpeas
- quarter cup fresh cilantro (sliced)
- 1 half cups frozen peas
- 4 scallions (thinly sliced)
- 1 red onion (thinly sliced)
- 1 red bell pepper (thinly sliced)
- 1 lime (halved)
- 3 garlic cloves (crushed)
- 1 small head cauliflower (bite-size florets)
- 3 tbsps red curry paste
- 1 tbsp extra-virgin olive oil
- Salt
- 1 tbsp fresh ginger (crushed)
- 1 tsp ground coriander
- Freshly ground black pepper
- 2 tsps chili powder

Instructions

Put the oil into a pan and heat it over moderate heat. For 5 mins, sauté the bell pepper and onion. Place the ginger and garlic in the dish. Add another minute to the sautéing. Include coriander, cauliflower, curry paste, and chili powder. Prepare for one minute. Add the coconut milk and heat through. Stir.

When the cauliflower is soft, remove it from the fire and discard the bay leaf. Lime juice should be added to the curry. Stir. Include the chickpeas and peas. Add some salt and pepper for flavor. Just let it a few mins to boil. Drizzle a spoonful of scallions and parsley over each serving. Serve.

Nutrition Calories: 442 Kcal, Proteins: 15g, Fat: 12g, Carbohydrates: 33g

3.8 Butternut Squash Carrot Soup

Preparation time: 20 Mins **Cooking time:** 15 Mins **Serving:** 4 Persons

Ingredients

- 1 pound of carrots (sliced)
- 1 half pounds of butternut squash (skinned and sliced)
- 4 cups vegetable stock
- 1 can coconut milk (full-fat)
- half cup shallots (sliced)
- 1 tsp salt
- 2 tbsps avocado oil
- Freshly ground black pepper
- 1 tbsp fresh ginger (grated)

Garnishing:

- Roasted chickpeas
- Coconut milk
- Cilantro

Instructions

Turn the oven temperature up to 400 degrees F. Spread parchment paper on a baking pan. Scatter the carrots, butternut squash, and shallots on the prepared baking sheet. Add oil and drizzle. Add some salt. Give the veggies a little toss to coat. Put them in the oven for 30 mins at 375 degrees. Give them a few mins to calm off. Mix the roasted veggies, vegetable stock, coconut milk, ginger, salt, and pepper in a mixer. Creamy consistency may be achieved by mixing. Put some soup in each of the four containers. Top each serving with chickpeas, coconut milk, and cilantro.

Nutrition Calories: 129 Kcal, Proteins: 6.5g, Fat: 2.7g, Carbohydrates: 23g

3.9 Kale Quinoa Shrimp Container

Preparation time: 25 Mins **Cooking time:** 30 Mins **Serving:** 4 Persons

Ingredients

Quinoa:

- 1 quarter cups quinoa
- 2 cups chicken broth
- Salt
- 2 tsps extra-virgin olive oil
- Freshly ground pepper

Kale:

- 2 tbsps extra-virgin olive oil
- Salt
- 1 bunch lacinato kale (roughly torn)
- Freshly ground black pepper

Shrimp and Toppings:

- 2 watermelon radishes (thinly sliced)
- 1 pound shrimp (skinned and deveined)
- 2 avocados (sliced)
- 1 tbsp extra-virgin olive oil
- 2 tbsps hot sauce
- 3/4 tsp ground coriander
- Salt
- Freshly ground black pepper
- 1 tsp ground cumin

Instructions

Quinoa: Put the olive oil in a saucepan and heat it over moderate heat. Mix in the quinoa and mix well. Toasted for one minute. Add to the stock. The quinoa has to boil till it is cooked. Add some salt and pepper for flavor.

Kale: Turn the oven temperature up to 400 degrees F. Use parchment paper to line a baking sheet. Mix the olive oil and kale together in a big mixing container. Add some salt and pepper for flavor. Mix by tossing. Toss the kale with the olive oil and spread it out in a thin layer on the baking sheet. For extra-crispy results, roast for fifteen mins.

Shrimp and Toppings: Olive oil should be heated in a pan over moderate heat. Toss the shrimp with the cumin, coriander, spicy sauce, salt, and pepper in a mixing dish. Mix by tossing. Heat a pan over moderate-high heat and sauté the shrimp mixture for 5 mins. Distribute the quinoa among four serving dishes. Crispy kale, avocado slices, watermelon radishes, and shrimp provide a delicious topping for the soup. Serve.

Nutrition Calories: 377 Kcal, Proteins: 37g, Fat: 7g, Carbohydrates: 436g

3.10 Egg Container and Veggies

Preparation time: 15 Mins **Cooking time:** 05 Mins **Serving:** 4 Persons

Ingredients

- 1 pound Brussels sprouts (cut in half)
- 1 pound sweet potatoes (diced)
- 4 eggs (poached)
- 1 half tbsps olive oil
- 3 tbsps apple cider vinegar
- 2 cups arugula
- 2 tbsps harissa

Instructions

Turn on the oven and set the temperature to 450 degrees F. Use parchment paper to line a baking sheet. Drizzle the Brussels sprouts and sweet potatoes evenly over the prepared baking sheet. Swirl in some olive oil. Add some salt and pepper for flavor. Cook at 400°F for 20 mins, or till meat is tender. Mix the harissa, olive oil, and apple cider vinegar in a separate container. Divvy up the roasted veggies into 4 serving dishes. Scatter arugula, harissa, and an egg dressing on each container. Serve.

Nutrition Calories: 263 Kcal, Proteins: 16g, Fat: 20g, Carbohydrates: 4.6g

3.11 Turkey Taco Containers

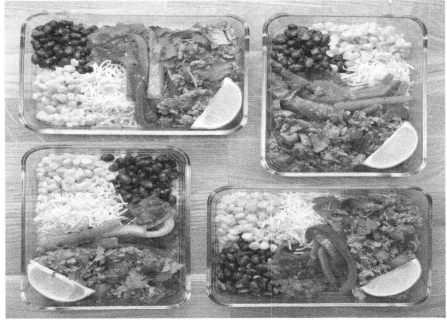

Preparation time: 20 Mins **Cooking time:** 15 Mins **Serving:** 2 Persons

Ingredients

Turkey:

- 2/3 cup water
- 3/4 pound ground turkey (lean)
- 2 tbsps taco seasoning

Salsa:

- quarter cup red onion (finely sliced)
- 1-pint cherry tomatoes (halved)
- 1 jalapeno (finely sliced)
- half lime (juiced)
- one-eighth tsp salt

Rice:

- 3/4 cup brown rice (uncooked)
- one-eighth tsp salt
- 1 lime (zested)

Topping:

- 1 can (12 oz.) of corn kernels (drained)

- half cup mozzarella (shredded)

Instructions

Follow the package directions for cooking the brown rice. It's as simple as seasoning the boiling water with salt and lime zest. Put the hot rice in a separate container to cool down. Put the turkey into a skillet and cook it over moderate heat. Leave the turkey in the oven for 10 mins, or till it's no pinker inside. Add the water and taco seasoning to the pot. Mix components by stirring. Keep the pot on low heat for two min to smooth the sauce. Put the turkey in a container of ice water. Put all the salsa components into a big mixing container. Throw everything together in a container and toss. Divide the rice among 4 serving dishes. Turkey and salsa may be used as toppings for the rice containers. Scatter the corn kernels and mozzarella over the top. Serve.

Nutrition Calories: 580 Kcal, Proteins: 26g, Fat: 25g, Carbohydrates: 62g

3.12 Bulgur Kale Pesto Salad

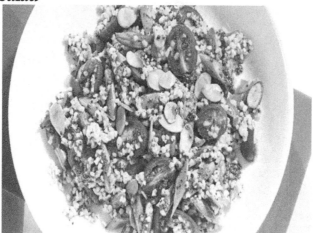

Preparation time: 10 Mins **Cooking time:** 05 Mins **Serving:** 2 Persons

Ingredients

- 1 half cups bulgur
- half pound of green beans
- half cup packed basil leaves
- quarter cup plus 3 tbsps almonds (toasted)
- 1 cup lacinato kale (thinly sliced)
- quarter cup lemon juice
- 1-pint grape tomatoes (halved)
- quarter cup extra-virgin olive oil
- quarter packed flat-leaf parsley
- 3 tbsps almonds (sliced)
- 1 garlic clove
- 1 tsp kosher salt (divided)
- half tsp kosher salt
- quarter tsp ground black pepper

Instructions

Place the garlic cloves in the container of a food processor. Chop it up in the food processor.

Add the almonds, basil, parsley, and kale. Pulse it till it's finely sliced. Add the lime juice, pepper, and a half tsp of salt. Mix everything up till it's silky smooth. Pesto is poured into bulgur. Incorporate the leftover toasted almonds, the green beans, and the tomatoes. Toss. Drizzle some sliced almonds on top. Serve.

Nutrition Calories: 218 Kcal, Proteins: 5.6g, Fat: 14g, Carbohydrates: 18g

3.13 Turkish Scrambled Eggs
Preparation time: 08 Mins **Cooking time:** 05 Mins **Serving:** 4 Persons

Ingredients

- 4 ripe tomatoes (diced)
- 6 eggs (beaten)
- 4 whole grain pitas (serving)
- 2 tbsps olive oil
- 3 scallions (finely sliced)
- Green olives (garnish)
- 2 tbsps fresh parsley (sliced)
- 4 oz. Feta cheese (crumbled)
- 2 big red bell peppers (seeded and finely sliced)
- 1 tsp red pepper flakes (crushed)
- quarter tsp ground black pepper
- half tsp kosher salt

Instructions

The oil should be heated in a pan on moderate heat. The scallions need two mins of cooking time to soften in the pan. Place the peppers inside. Stir-fry for five mins. The tomatoes and pepper flakes should be added now. Add another five mins of sautéing. Toss in some eggs and cheese. Shake and mix incessantly to create a scramble. The eggs need to be cooked through. Add some salt and pepper for flavor. Remove the heat source. Include the sliced parsley in the mixture. Spread olives on top. Pitas should be served on the side.

Nutrition Calories: 240 Kcal, Proteins: 12g, Fat: 14g, Carbohydrates: 19g

3.14 Swiss Chard and Red Lentil Curried Soup
Preparation time: 18 Mins **Cooking time:** 10 Mins **Serving:** 4 Persons

Ingredients

- 2 cups dried red lentils
- 1 pound Swiss chard
- 5 cups vegetable broth
- 6 tbsps thick Greek yogurt
- 1 can (15 oz.) of chickpeas (rinsed and drained)
- 5 tsps curry powder
- 1 big onion (thinly sliced)

- 2 tbsps olive oil
- 1 lime (sliced into 6 wedges)
- quarter tsp ground cayenne pepper
- 1 red jalapeño chili (stemmed and thinly sliced)
- 1 tsp salt

Instructions

Put the oil in a pot and heat it over moderate heat. When the onion is soft and translucent, it's ready to be sautéed. Curry and cayenne pepper should be stirred in. Place the chard and Four cups of broth into the pot. Keep stirring at a boil till the chard is wilted, about 5 mins. Add the lentils and chickpeas and stir. Turn down the stove. Stir occasionally and cook at a low simmer for 18 mins or till lentils are tender. Get rid of the hot water or the heater. About 1/2 of the soup should be put in a food processor. Into a smooth consistency, of course. Return the puréed mixture to the cooking kettle. Add the rest of the salt and broth. Stir. Get the soup nice and toasty for a few mins on low heat. Distribute across 6 containers. Yogurt, a lime wedge, and sliced jalapenos make a great garnish. Serve.

Nutrition Calories: 169 Kcal, Proteins: 10g, Fat: 2.82g, Carbohydrates: 26g

3.15 Orange Cardamom Quinoa with Carrots

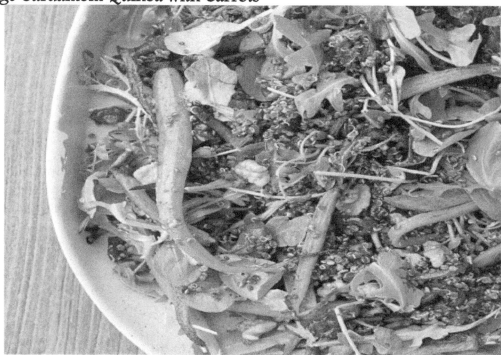

Preparation time: 15 Mins **Cooking time:** 0 Mins **Serving:** 4 Persons

Ingredients

- 2 half cups vegetable broth
- 1 pound of carrots (skinned and sliced)
- 1 cup quinoa (rinsed)
- 2 oranges (zested and segmented)
- one-third cup golden raisins
- 1-inch fresh ginger (skinned and crushed)

- 1 tsp ground cardamom
- half tsp freshly ground black pepper
- half tsp salt

Instructions

The orange zest, salt, black pepper, cardamom, raisins, ginger, carrots, quinoa, and broth go into the slow cooker. Combo together successfully. For a low and slow cooking time of three and a half hrs, start this. Evenly disperse the quinoa between 4 serving dishes. Add a few orange segments on the top of each serving. Serve.

Nutrition Calories: 170 Kcal, Proteins: 5g, Fat: 3g, Carbohydrates: 31g

3.16 Quinoa Turmeric Power Container
Preparation time: 15 Mins **Cooking time:** 30 Mins **Serving:** 4 Persons

Ingredients

- 2 kale leaves (rinsed)
- 7 small yellow potatoes (slice into strips)
- 1 avocado (sliced)
- 1 can (15 oz.) of chickpeas (drained and rinsed)
- Pepper
- quarter cup quinoa
- 1 tbsp coconut oil
- 1 tsp paprika
- Salt
- half tbsp olive oil
- 2 tsps turmeric(divided)

Instructions

Turn the oven temperature up to 360 degrees Fahrenheit. Place the potato strips flat on half of the baking sheet. Coconut oil should be drizzled over the top. Add some salt, pepper, and turmeric (about a tsp's worth) for seasoning. Keep turning after 5 mins. Put the paprika and chickpeas in a big container and mix well. Mix well by tossing. On the opposite side of the baking sheet, separate the chickpeas from the potatoes. Toss in the oven and set the timer for 25 mins. Put half a cup of liquid and the quinoa in a saucepan and cook it on low to moderate heat. Let the quinoa simmer till it's soft. Spice it up with a tweak of of turmeric, some pepper, and salt. Mix well. Putting it aside to cool is a good idea. The kale benefits from a massage with olive oil. Split the leaves between 4 serving dishes. Arrange quinoa, avocado slices, and roasted veggies in separate containers. Serve.

Nutrition Calories: 470 Kcal, Proteins: 14g, Fat: 17g, Carbohydrates: 72g

3.17 Tomato Stew with Chickpea and Kale
Preparation time: 15 Mins **Cooking time:** 20 Mins **Serving:** 4 Persons

Ingredients

- 3/4 pound kale (stemmed and leaves coarsely sliced)
- 1 pound of tomatoes (cored and sliced)

- 1 cup vegetable stock

- 1 moderate onion (sliced into eighths)

- 2 cans (15-ounce) chickpeas (drained and rinsed)

- 6 garlic cloves (thinly sliced)

- quarter tsp red pepper flakes (crushed)

- 4 tbsps olive oil (divided)

- 4 big eggs

- 1 quarter tsp kosher salt (divided)

Instructions

A quarter of the oil should be heated in a pan on moderate heat. Coupling the onion with a quarter of the salt is the first step. In a skillet, heat the oil and cook the onions for 10 mins. Add the crushed red pepper and crushed garlic and stir. Keep cooking for another two mins. Include the kale. Get it as soft as possible by cooking it. Add the canned tomatoes, chickpeas, and chicken stock. Prepare in ten mins. Just add salt. Put the rest of the oil in a pan and heat it over moderate heat. Prepare an egg by cracking it open and cooking it till the white is done and the bottom becomes crunchy. Repeat with the rest of the eggs. Create 4 containers and equally distribute the stew. Add an egg on top. Just add salt. Serve.

Nutrition Calories: 212 Kcal, Proteins: 6.4g, Fat: 5.1g, Carbohydrates: 37g

3.18 Anti-Inflammatory Beef Meatballs
Preparation time: 10 Mins **Cooking time:** 10 Mins **Serving:** 4 Persons

Ingredients

- quarter cup sliced cilantro (tightly packed)

- 2 pounds of ground beef

- half tsp ground ginger

- Zest of 1 lime

- half tsp sea salt

- 5 garlic cloves (pressed)

Instructions

Turn on the oven and set the temperature to 350 degrees F. Put parchment paper on a baking sheet. Put everything you need in a basin and mix it together. Maintain a healthy mix. Make 12 meatballs from the mixture. Line a baking sheet with foil and distribute the meatballs on it. Put it in the oven and set the timer for 25 mins. You may garnish the meatballs with fresh herbs and avocado slices.

Nutrition Calories: 57 Kcal, Proteins: 4g, Fat: 7g, Carbohydrates: 3g

3.19 Salmon with Veggies Sheet Pan
Preparation time: 20 Mins **Cooking time:** 30 Mins **Serving:** 4 Persons

Ingredients

- 16 oz. bag of baby potatoes

- 1 tsp fresh thyme

- 16 oz. Brussels sprouts (halved)

- 4 6-ounce salmon fillets (skin on)
- 1 cup cherry tomatoes
- half red onion (cubed)
- 1 bunch of asparagus (trimmed and halved)
- 3 tbsps balsamic vinegar
- 1 garlic clove (crushed)
- 2 tbsps honey
- 1 tbsp Dijon mustard
- 2 tbsps olive oil
- half tsp sea salt

Instructions

Prepare a 450 F oven temperature. Prepare parchment paper on a baking pan. To make the dressing, mix the vinegar, garlic, honey, Dijon mustard, thyme, and salt in a container. Maintain a healthy mix. Asparagus, red onion, Brussels sprouts, potatoes, tomatoes, olive oil, and three tbsps. The balsamic honey combination should be mixd in a separate container. Maintain a healthy mix. Prepare a baking sheet by spreading the veggies equally over it. Put in the oven for 10 mins. The oven is done, so remove it. Salmon fillets should be arranged atop the veggies. It's skin-side down. Apply the rest of the balsamic honey mixture to each fillet by brushing it on. The baking sheet should be returned to the oven. Put in the oven for 10 mins. For the next four mins, broil on high. The fillets' exposed surfaces will brown in this manner. Serve.

Nutrition Calories: 377 Kcal, Proteins: 38g, Fat: 10g, Carbohydrates: 39g

3.20 Roasted Salmon Garlic and Broccoli

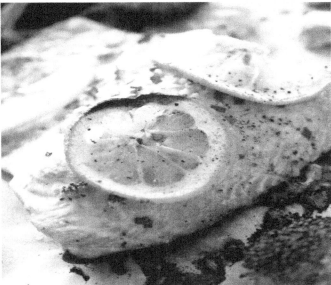

Preparation time: 25 Mins **Cooking time:** 35 Mins **Serving:** 4 Persons

Ingredients

- 1 lemon (sliced)
- 1 half pounds salmon fillets
- 1 big broccoli head (sliced into florets)
- 2 half tbsps coconut oil (melted and divided)

- 3/4 tsp sea salt (divided)
- 2 cloves fresh garlic (crushed)
- Black pepper

Instructions

Prepare a 450 F oven temperature. Put parchment paper on a baking sheet. Put the salmon in an even layer on the prepared baking sheet. There has to be breathing room between the various components. A tsp of olive oil should be used to finish cooking the salmon. Distribute the garlic cloves in a thin layer over the fish. Add ½ of the salt and enough pepper as required. Place a lemon slice atop each serving of fish. Putting aside. Place the broccoli florets, rest of the pepper, salt, and one and a half tsps of oil in a mixing basin and toss to mix. Toss. Florets should be placed between each slice of salmon. Put the dish in the oven, and set the timer for fifteen min. Parsley and lemon wedges make a lovely garnish. Serve.

Nutrition Calories: 366 Kcal, Proteins: 35g, Fat: 14g, Carbohydrates: 29g

3.21 Roasted Sweet Potatoes with Avocado Dip
Preparation time: 25 Mins **Cooking time:** 40 Mins **Serving:** 4 Persons

Ingredients

- 1 avocado (halved and pitted)
- 2 big sweet potatoes (washed and cubed)
- 1 lime (juice)
- 4 tbsps water
- 1 big clove of garlic (skinned and sliced)
- half tsp sea salt (divided)
- 1 tsp olive oil
- 2 tbsps olive oil

Instructions

Turn the oven temperature up to 400 degrees F. Use parchment paper to line a baking sheet. Place the diced potatoes in an equal layer on the prepared baking sheet. Use 2 tbsp of olive oil to drizzle. To ensure that all of the potato pieces get a coating of oil, you should turn them over. Use a third of the salt for seasoning. Put it in the oven for 40-45 mins, or till it's a golden brown. Put the avocados, garlic, lime juice, and the rest of the half of the salt in a mixer and mix till smooth. Mix till the point of smoothness. Stir in the olive oil and the water gradually. Make sure everything is well mixed by continuing to mix. Prepare a dip to accompany the cooked potatoes and serve.

Nutrition Calories: 188 Kcal, Proteins: 3g, Fat: 13g, Carbohydrates: 20g

3.22 Chicken with Lemon and Asparagus
Preparation time: 15 Mins **Cooking time:** 20 Mins **Serving:** 4 Persons

Ingredients

- 2 cups asparagus (sliced)
- 1 pound of chicken breasts (boneless and skinless)
- quarter cup flour
- 2 lemons (sliced)

- 4 tbsps butter (divided)
- 1 tsp lemon pepper seasoning
- half tsp salt
- half tsp pepper

Instructions

Lemons and Asparagus: The rest of the butter should be melted in the same pan over moderate heat. Pour in the asparagus. Heat till the vegetables are crisp-tender. Remove from the stove. Place the lemon slices in a single layer on the hot skillet. Caramelization is achieved by cooking for a few mins on each side without stirring. Remove from the stovetop.

Chicken: To make slices that are just 3/4 of an inch thick, cut each chicken chest in half lengthwise. Put the flour, salt, and pepper into a wide, shallow dish. Mix in a harmonious manner. Drizzle the flour mixture over each piece of chicken. Prepare the first half of the butter by melting it in a pan over moderate heat. Place the chicken pieces within. To get a golden brown color, cook for Five mins for each side. While cooking, season both sides of the chicken using lime pepper. Putting aside.

Assembly: Arrange the cooked asparagus, lemon, and chicken in tiers on a serving plate. Serve.

Nutrition Calories: 250 Kcal, Proteins: 13g, Fat: 7g, Carbohydrates: 26g

3.23 Lentil Soup with Lemons

Preparation time: 15 Mins **Cooking time:** 20 Mins **Serving:** 8 Persons

Ingredients

- 1 half cups celery (diced)
- 2 cups green lentils
- 1 half cups carrots (diced)
- 1 tbsp extra-virgin olive oil
- 2 half boxes (32 oz.) of vegetable broth
- 3 cloves garlic (crushed)
- 1 yellow onion (diced)
- Zest of half lemon
- 3 small lemons (juiced)
- 2 tsps dried turmeric
- 1 tsp salt
- 4 tsps fresh ginger (grated)

Instructions

Put the oil in a Dutch oven and heat it over moderate heat. Prepare the salt, onion, celery, and carrots in a sauté pan for 5 mins. Add the garlic and ginger and mix well. Keep cooking for another minute. Add the lentils, turmeric, and broth to a pot and mix well. Put the thermostat down a notch. Half-cover the pot and boil the soup for 45 mins. Mix with some fresh lime juice and zest. Mix. Add another 30 mins to the cooking time for the soup. Serve.

Nutrition Calories: 68 Kcal, Proteins: 5g, Fat: 0.5g, Carbohydrates: 12g

3.24 Shrimp Fajitas
Preparation time: 25 Mins **Cooking time:** 25 Mins **Serving:** 4 Persons

Ingredients

- 1 red bell pepper (sliced thinly)
- 1 half pounds of shrimp
- 1 yellow bell pepper
- 1 small red onion
- 1 orange bell pepper
- 1 half tbsps extra virgin olive oil
- 1 tsp kosher salt
- 2 tsps chili powder
- half tsp onion powder
- Fresh cilantro (for garnish)
- half tsp smoked paprika
- half tsp garlic powder
- half tsp ground cumin
- Lime
- Freshly ground pepper
- Tortillas (warmed)

Instructions

The oven should be warm uped at 450 degrees F. Spray cooking spray onto a baking sheet. Put the shrimp, peppers, onions, spices, olive oil, and salt into a big mixing container. Make sure to give it a good toss. Distribute them in a single layer on the baking sheet. Put in oven and bake for 10 min. Go ahead and turn the oven to broil. To finish cooking the fajita, wait 2 mins. Lime juice should be squeezed over the fajita. Use cilantro as a garnish. Put on heated tortillas and serve.

Nutrition Calories: 241 Kcal, Proteins: 14g, Fat: 10g, Carbohydrates: 25g

3.25 Mediterranean One Pan Cod
Preparation time: 15 Mins **Cooking time:** 20 Mins **Serving:** 4 Persons

Ingredients

- 2 cups fennel (sliced)
- 2 cups kale (shredded)
- 1 cup fresh tomatoes (diced)
- half cup water
- 1 cup oil-cured black olives
- 1 pound cod (quartered)
- 1 can (14.5 oz.) diced tomato
- 1 small onion (sliced)

- 3 big cloves of garlic (sliced)
- Pinch of red pepper (crushed)
- 1 tsp orange zest
- 2 tbsps olive oil
- half tsp dried oregano
- quarter tsp black pepper
- quarter tsp fennel seeds
- one-eighth tsp salt

Garnish:
- Orange zest
- Fresh oregano
- Fennel fronds
- Olive oil

Instructions

The olive oil should be heated in a pan over moderate heat. Fennel, onion, and garlic should be cooked together for 8 mins. You may add salt and pepper as required. Incorporate the tinned tomatoes, water, fresh tomatoes, and kale. Just add 12 additional mins of cooking time. Add the oregano, pepper, and olives, and stir to mix. Toss the fish with a mixture of pepper, fennel seeds, salt, and lemon or lime juice. Place the fish fillets in the tomato sauce. Tightly cover the skillet. Ten mins at a low simmer. Garnish. Serve.

Nutrition Calories: 333 Kcal, Proteins: 43g, Fat: 10g, Carbohydrates: 19g

3.26 Garlic Tomato Basil Chicken

Preparation time: 20 Mins **Cooking time:** 15 Mins **Serving:** 4 Persons

Ingredients
- 4 moderate zucchini (spiralized)
- 1 pound of chicken breasts (boneless and skinless)
- Salt
- 1 cup fresh basil (loosely packed and cut into ribbons)
- 3 garlic cloves (crushed)
- Pepper
- 14.5-ounce can of sliced tomatoes
- half yellow onion (diced)
- quarter tsp red pepper flakes (crushed)
- 2 tbsps olive oil (divided)

Instructions

Use plastic wrap to enclose each chicken breast. Beat them to a uniform thickness of one inch. Tear open each chicken breast. You may add salt and pepper as required. Place a tsp of olive oil in a pan and heat it over moderate heat. Chicken breasts should be placed. Brown them in a pan and cook them all the way through. Putting aside. Put the leftover olive oil in the same pan and heat it over moderate. Keep the onion cooking for around 5 mins, and add the garlic. Keep sautéing for another minute. Add the tomatoes and basil and mix well. Add some crushed red pepper, black pepper, and salt as required. Put it on low heat and mix it every so often for 10 mins. Mix in the chicken breasts and zoodles. Allow to heat slowly for a couple of moments. Serve.

Nutrition Calories: 686 Kcal, Proteins: 34g, Fat: 40g, Carbohydrates: 46g

3.27 Asian Garlic Noodles

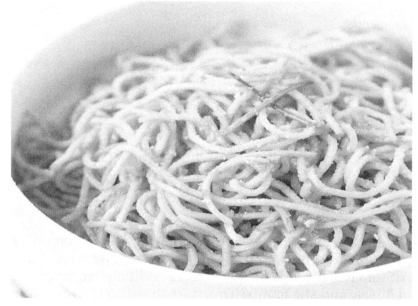

Preparation time: 05 Mins **Cooking time:** 10 Mins **Serving:** 4 Persons

Ingredients

Noodles:

- 1 small red bell pepper (crushed)
- 1 big spaghetti squash
- half cup fresh cilantro (diced)
- half big carrot (julienne cut)
- quarter cup roasted cashews (sliced)
- half moderate zucchini (julienne cut)

Sauce:

- 6 garlic cloves
- 6 big Medjool dates (pitted)
- 2 tbsps fish sauce
- quarter cup coconut milk (full fat)
- 2 tbsps red curry paste
- 2/3 cup coconut aminos
- 2 tbsps fresh ginger (grated)

Instructions

Please warm up your oven to 425 degrees F. Make a horizontal cut across the spaghetti squash. Remove the pulp by scraping it. Arrange the spaghetti squash cut-side up on a baking sheet.

Olive oil should be brushed over the exposed area. Set the oven timer for 30 min. A noodle-like texture may be achieved by scraping the flesh with a fork. To make the sauce, throw all the components into a mixer. Puree. Throw all the noodle-making stuff into a container and mix it together. Cover the noodles with the sauce. Mix in a harmonious manner. Serve.

Nutrition Calories: 426 Kcal, Proteins: 30g, Fat: 7g, Carbohydrates: 62g

3.28 Shrimp Garlic Zoodles
Preparation time: 15 Mins **Cooking time:** 05 Mins **Serving:** 4 Persons

Ingredients

- 2 moderate zucchini
- 3/4 pounds moderate shrimp
- 4 cloves garlic (crushed)
- Salt
- Red pepper flakes
- 1 tbsp olive oil
- Zest and juice of 1 lemon
- Fresh parsley (sliced)
- Pepper

Instructions

Cook the zoodles in a spiralizer set to moderate. Putting aside. Stir the olive oil, lime zest, and lime juice together in a pan over moderate heat. The shrimp should be added and stirred in. Keep it in the oven for a couple of mins. Put the crushed red pepper and garlic in a container and stir them in. Keep cooking for another minute. Start cooking the zoodles. Three mins of tossing should be enough time to get a moderate-rare consistency. You may add salt and pepper as required. Dress with sliced parsley. Serve.

Nutrition Calories: 286 Kcal, Proteins: 27g, Fat: 5.7g, Carbohydrates: 8.1g

3.29 Cauliflower Grits and Shrimp
Preparation time: 15 Mins **Cooking time:** 05 Mins **Serving:** 4 Persons

Ingredients

Cauliflower Grits:

- 1 big clove of garlic (sliced)
- 1 bag (12 oz.) of frozen cauliflower
- Salt
- 2 tbsps butter

Shrimp:

- 3 tbsps Cajun seasoning (no salt)
- 1 pound big shrimp (skinned and deveined)
- 2 tbsps butter
- Salt

Instructions

The cauliflower and the garlic should be steamed together in a pot. Waiting to be steamed till soft. (The piping hot liquid should not be thrown away). Put the garlic, steamed cauliflower, and butter in a food processor. The consistency may be adjusted throughout processing. If you want a thinner or thicker consistency, add additional hot water and salt and mix again. Putting aside. Mix the Cajun seasonings in a container. Sprinkling the spice on the shrimp is not enough. Put some salt on it. Butter should be melted in a pan over moderate heat. Add the shrimp. Cook till the internal temperature of the meat reaches 160 F. Divide the grits into 2 containers and top with the cauliflower. Place the shrimp on top once they have been cooked. When serving, transfer the gravy from the pan to the containers. Serve.

Nutrition Calories: 350 Kcal, Proteins: 37g, Fat: 16g, Carbohydrates: 21g

3.30 Green Curry

Preparation time: 20 Mins **Cooking time:** 15 Mins **Serving:** 4 Persons

Ingredients

- 12 oz. tofu (firm)
- 3 cups broccoli florets
- A swish of olive oil
- 3 cans (14 oz.) of coconut milk
- 2 sweet potatoes (skinned and cubed)
- 4 tbsps green curry paste
- A drizzle of salt

Garnish:

- Fresh cilantro (sliced)
- Fish sauce
- Golden raisins
- Brown sugar

Instructions

Use towels to rinse the tofu. Cube the tofu and set it aside. Put the olive oil in a pan and warm it over moderate heat. Toss the tofu in the pan. Put some salt on it. Cook the tofu in hot oil for fifteen min, occasionally turning till it is golden brown all over. Putting aside. Mix the curry paste, coconut milk, and sweet potatoes in the same saucepan and heat over moderate. Hold at a low boil for ten mins. Add the broccoli and tofu to the pan. Simmer for another 5 mins. Flourish. Serve.

Nutrition Calories: 328 Kcal, Proteins: 24g, Fat: 20g, Carbohydrates: 17g

CHAPTER 4: Anti-Inflammatory Dinner Recipes

4.1 Stir-Fried Snap Pea and Chicken

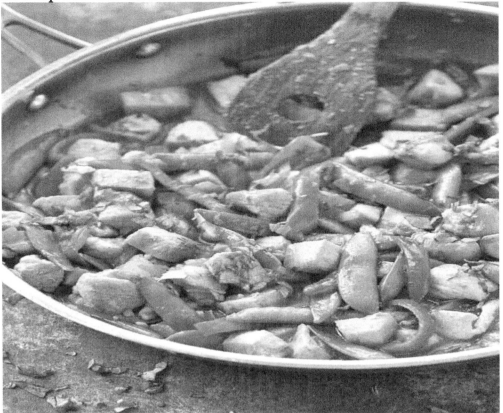

Preparation time: 20 Mins **Cooking time:** 15 Mins **Serving:** 4 Persons

Ingredients

- 2 half cups snap peas
- 1 quarter cups chicken breast (skinless, boneless, and sliced thinly)
- 1 bunch of scallions (sliced thinly)
- 2 tbsps vegetable oil
- 1 red bell pepper (sliced thinly)
- 3 tbsps fresh cilantro
- 2 tbsps sesame seeds (+ more for garnish)
- 3 tbsps soy sauce
- 2 tbsps rice vinegar
- Freshly ground black pepper
- 2 garlic cloves (crushed)
- Salt
- 2 tsps Sriracha

Instructions

Put the oil in a pan and heat it over moderate heat. The scallions and garlic should be sautéed for a minute. Cooked snap peas and red bell pepper should be added to the pot. Add some oil and saute for three mins. Drop the chicken in there. Add another 5 mins of cooking time.

Mix the rice vinegar, sesame seeds, soy sauce, and Sriracha. Put everything in a container and mix it together. Wait 2 mins while it simmers. Incorporate the sliced cilantro. Stir. Drizzle some sesame seeds and sliced cilantro over each dish. Serve.

Nutrition Calories: 261 Kcal, Proteins: 29g, Fat: 10g, Carbohydrates: 14g

4.2 Turkey Chili with Avocado

Preparation time: 25 Mins **Cooking time:** 22 Mins **Serving:** 8 Persons

Ingredients

- 4 cups chicken broth
- 1 pound ground turkey
- 1 can (15 oz.) of white beans
- 1 big white onion (diced)
- 1 can (15 oz.) of corn kernels
- 1 avocado (diced)
- Freshly ground black pepper
- 2 tbsps extra-virgin olive oil
- 4 garlic cloves (crushed)
- 2 tsps ground cumin
- 1 tsp ground coriander
- 1 tsp cayenne pepper
- Salt

Instructions

Put the olive oil in a pan and warm it over moderate flame. Put the onion in a pan and cook it for 8 mins. Mix in the garlic. Maintain the low heat for one more min of sauteing. Place the turkey inside. To ensure thorough cooking, set the timer for 7 mins. Spice it up with cayenne, cumin, coriander, pepper, and salt. Stir. Maintain heat for a few mins. Add the broth to the pot. The components should be left to cook at a low simmer for 35 mins. Prepare the maize and beans. Keep at a low boil for a further 3 mins. Add some sliced avocado to the top of each dish. Serve.

Nutrition Calories: 686 Kcal, Proteins: 47g, Fat: 46g, Carbohydrates: 14g

4.3 Turkey Burgers with Tzatziki Sauce

Preparation time: 22 Mins **Cooking time:** 20 Mins **Serving:** 4 Persons

Ingredients

- half cup fresh parsley (sliced)
- 1 pound ground turkey
- 3/4 cup bread crumbs
- 1 egg
- 1 sweet onion (crushed)
- 2 garlic cloves (crushed)
- quarter tsp red-pepper flakes

- 1 tbsp extra-virgin olive oil
- half tsp dried oregano
- Salt
- Freshly ground black pepper

Tzatziki Sauce:

- 1 cup Greek yogurt
- half European cucumber (diced)
- quarter cup fresh parsley (sliced)
- 1 tbsp extra-virgin olive oil
- 2 tbsps lemon juice
- 1 tweak of of garlic powder
- Salt
- Freshly ground black pepper

Toppings:

- half red onion (sliced)
- 4 hamburger buns (whole-wheat)
- 8 Boston lettuce leaves
- 2 tomatoes (sliced)

Instructions

Burgers: Put the oil in a pan and heat it over moderate heat. For around 4 mins, saute the onion. Add the garlic. Maintain the low heat for one more min of sauteing. Putting aside. Mix the turkey, oregano, pepper flakes, parsley, cooled onion, and egg in a big mixing basin. Mix in a harmonious manner. Add the bread crumbs, seasoning, and pepper. Mix in a harmonious manner. Turn the oven temperature up to 350 degrees F. Make 4 burgers out of the turkey mixture. Put some cooking spray in a skillet that can go from the stovetop to the oven and heat it over moderate. Place the burger inside. Brown the meat by searing it for 5 mins on each side. You should bake the skillet. The burgers need to be baked for 17 mins.

Tzatziki Sauce: Put the garlic powder, olive oil, lime juice, yogurt, and cucumber in a container and stir well. Mix in a harmonious manner. You may add salt and pepper as required. The parsley should be added now.

Nutrition Calories: 350 Kcal, Proteins: 54g, Fat: 7g, Carbohydrates: 10g

4.4 Fried Rice with Pineapple

Preparation time: 10 Mins **Cooking time:** 15 Mins **Serving:** 3 Persons

Ingredients

- half cup frozen corn
- 3 cups brown rice (cooked)
- 2 cups pineapple (diced)
- half cup ham (diced)
- half cup frozen peas

- 3 tbsps soy sauce
- 1 tbsp sesame oil
- 2 tbsps olive oil
- 2 green onions (sliced)
- 1 onion (diced)
- 2 carrots (skinned and grated)
- 2 cloves garlic (crushed)
- half tsp ginger powder
- quarter tsp white pepper

Instructions

Mix the soy sauce, sesame oil, ginger powder, and white ginger powder in a container. Mix in a harmonious manner. The olive oil should be heated in a pan over moderate heat. For around 4 mins, sauté the onion and garlic. Coat the pan with oil and add the vegetables. Prepare in 4 mins. Add the rice, pineapple, ham, green onions, and soy sauce mixture to the pan. Continue stirring for a few mins as the food cooks. Serve.

Nutrition Calories: 179 Kcal, Proteins: 3g, Fat: 5g, Carbohydrates: 30g

4.5 Ratatouille

Preparation time: 10 Mins **Cooking time:** 15 Mins **Serving:** 5 Persons

Ingredients

- 1 moderate red onion (thickly sliced)
- 1 small eggplant
- 1 cup tomato sauce
- 2 small red bell peppers (halved)
- 2 moderate summer squash
- Salt
- 2 moderate zucchini
- 3 moderate tomatoes
- 2 sprigs oregano
- 2 garlic cloves (smashed)
- Freshly ground black pepper
- 2 tbsps thyme leaves
- 5 tbsps olive oil

Instructions

Turn the oven temperature up to 375 degrees F. Prepare a baking tray for four individual plates. Put the oil in a saucepan and heat it over moderate heat. Garlic should be cooked for a minute in a skillet. Shut off the furnace. Mix in the oregano. Wait 15 mins and strain. Throw out the oregano and garlic. Put 2 tbsps of the oil into each individual baking dish. Apply a little amount of tomato sauce to the bottom of each baking tray. Distribute the eggplant, squash, onion, zucchini, tomato, and bell pepper evenly among the baking dishes. Slices should be closely packed and slightly staggered. Add the rest of the tomato sauce and spread it out. Use the leftover olive oil as a finishing touch. Add thyme, pepper, and salt as required. Do a 30-minute roast. Give it a few mins to cool off. Serve.

Nutrition Calories: 127 Kcal, Proteins: 2.1g, Fat: 7.1g, Carbohydrates: 16g

4.6 Eggs with Tomatoes and Asparagus
Preparation time: 10 Mins **Cooking time:** 10 Mins **Serving:** 4 Persons

Ingredients

- 2 pounds asparagus
- 1-pint cherry tomatoes
- 4 eggs
- Salt
- 2 tbsps olive oil
- 2 tsps fresh thyme (sliced)
- Pepper

Instructions

Turn the oven temperature up to 400 degrees F. Spray some cooking spray in a baking dish.

Arrange a single layer of tomato halves and asparagus spears on the oiled baking sheet. Spread the olive oil throughout. Spice it up with salt, pepper, and thyme. Cook at 400° for 12 mins. Take it out of the oven. Make an omelet with the asparagus and the eggs. Add salt and pepper as required. Put the dish in the oven and set the timer for 7 mins. Serve.

Nutrition Calories: 290 Kcal, Proteins: 13g, Fat: 17g, Carbohydrates: 21g

4.7 Turmeric, Carrot, and Ginger Soup
Preparation time: 10 Mins **Cooking time:** 10 Mins **Serving:** 4 Persons

Ingredients

- 3 carrots (diced)
- 4 cups vegetable stock
- Canned coconut milk (for topping)
- 3 cloves garlic (crushed)
- 1-inch fresh ginger (finely grated)
- 2 inches of fresh turmeric (finely grated)
- 1 white onion (diced)
- Black sesame seeds (for topping)
- 1 tbsp lemon juice

Instructions

Put some olive oil in a saucepan and cook it over moderate heat. Caramelize the onion in a skillet. Prepare the dish by adding the spices. Keep cooking for another minute. Prepare by adding carrots. To prepare, you will need to spend two mins cooking. Incorporate the vegetable stock. Maintain a low boil for 25 mins. Use a stick mixer to purée the soup. Prepare the dish by adding lemon juice. Stir.

To serve, stir with some coconut milk and drizzle with black sesame seeds.

Nutrition Calories: 103 Kcal, Proteins: 2g, Fat: 3g, Carbohydrates: 18g

---

4.8 Bulgur and Sweet Potato Salad
Preparation time: 15 Mins **Cooking time:** 40 Mins **Serving:** 4 Persons

Ingredients

- 1 quarter cups bulgur wheat
- 2 moderate sweet potatoes
- 1 cup parsley (finely sliced)
- quarter cup olive oil
- half cup mint (finely sliced)
- quarter cup red onion (finely sliced)
- 2 tbsps orange zest
- quarter cup orange juice (freshly squeezed)
- 2 tbsps lemon juice
- 1 tbsp avocado oil
- 1 tbsp red wine vinegar
- 2 tsps maple syrup
- 1 small clove of garlic (grated)
- half tsp salt
- Coarse salt
- Freshly ground black pepper
- Black pepper

Instructions

Turn on the oven to 450 degrees Fahrenheit. Prepare parchment paper on a baking pan. The sweet potatoes, maple syrup, and avocado oil should be mixed in a container. Add salt and pepper as required. Mix by tossing. Evenly disperse on the prepared baking sheet. Set the timer for 40 mins and roast. Toss during the midway point of roasting. Bring 3 and a half cups of water to a boil in a saucepan set over moderate heat. Start a boil with this. Add the bulgur to the pot. Stir. Turn down the stove. Stirring occasionally, let simmer for 8 mins. Shut off the furnace. Put the lid on it. Keep quiet for 10 mins. Get rid of the fluid. Gently stir the bulgur. Mix the garlic, pepper, vinegar, salt, citrus juices, olive oil, and orange juice in a container. Mix everything well. Mix the vinegar and garlic in a separate container; add the bulgur, parsley, mint, orange zest, and red onion. Mix by tossing. Serve.

Nutrition Calories: 103 Kcal, Proteins: 2g, Fat: 3g, Carbohydrates: 18g

4.9 Salmon Roast with Romaine and Potatoes

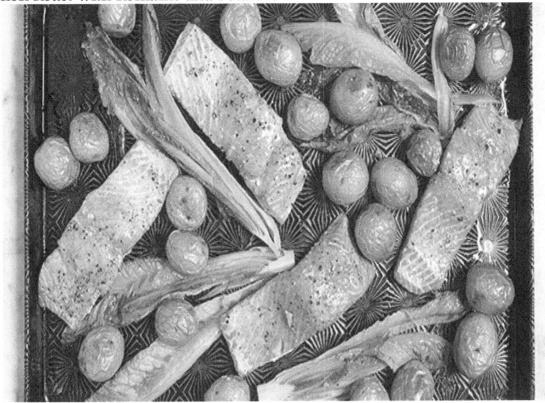

Preparation time: 15 Mins **Cooking time:** 30 Mins **Serving:** 4 Persons

Ingredients

- 2 hearts of romaine lettuce (cut in half)
- 1 pound of baby potatoes (rinsed)
- 4 (6-ounce) salmon fillets
- 1 tbsp butter (melted)
- 4 tbsps olive oil (divided)
- 1 tsp lemon juice
- Freshly ground black pepper
- quarter tsp paprika
- Salt

Instructions

Turn on the oven to 450 degrees F. Put some cooking spray on a baking sheet. Place the rest of the potatoes and olive oil in a container. Place on coat and toss. Put the potatoes in a single layer on a baking sheet that has been oiled. Roast for twenty mins at 400°. Mix the rest of the olive oil and the lime juice, and rub it into the romaine lettuce. Put some salt and pepper on it. The fillets of salmon should be brushed with melted butter. Drizzle with salt, pepper, and paprika. Salmon fillets, romaine lettuce, and potatoes should all be spread out on a baking pan. Repeat the roasting process for 7 more mins. Serve.

Nutrition Calories: 147 Kcal, Proteins: 0g, Fat: 4g, Carbohydrates: 1g

4.10 Bean Bolognese

Preparation time: 15 Mins **Cooking time:** 30 Mins **Serving:** 4 Persons

Ingredients

- 1 can (14-ounce) white beans
- 2 carrots (skinned and sliced)
- 1 moderate onion (sliced)
- 1 can (28-ounce) crushed tomatoes
- 2 cloves garlic (crushed)
- 2 celery stalks (sliced)

Instructions

Put everything into a slow cooker. Put it in the oven and let it there for 6 hrs. Serve.

Nutrition Calories: 442 Kcal, Proteins: 17g, Fat: 11g, Carbohydrates: 68g

4.11 Peppers Stuffed with Sweet Potato and Turkey

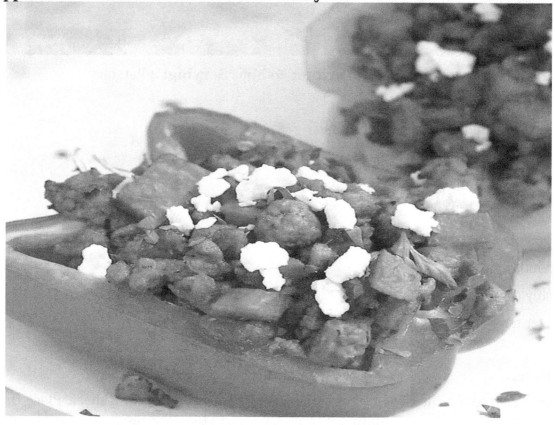

Preparation time: 15 Mins **Cooking time:** 20 Mins **Serving:** 4 Persons

Ingredients

- 1 2/3 cups sweet potatoes (diced)
- 2 cups ground turkey
- half cup tomato sauce
- 2 big bell peppers (cut in half)
- half cup onions (diced)

- 1 tbsp extra-virgin olive oil
- Pepper
- 2 cloves garlic (crushed)
- Fresh parsley (for garnishing)
- Salt

Instructions

Get the oven ready at 350 degrees. Spray some cooking spray on a baking sheet. Olive oil should be heated in a pan over moderate heat. Add the turkey and garlic. Break up the meat while it cooks and let it simmer for 10 mins while being stirred occasionally. Toss the onions in. You just need 5 mins to cook. Mix the potatoes into the mixture. Cover. Maintain a simmer for 8 mins, stirring occasionally. Mix in the salt, pepper, and tomato sauce. Put the peppers in a single layer on a prepared baking sheet. Here, the opening is pointing upwards. Stuff the sweet potato and turkey mixture into the bell peppers till they are almost full. Put in the oven and set the timer for 30 mins. Dress with sliced parsley. Serve.

Nutrition Calories: 324 Kcal, Proteins: 25g, Fat: 13g, Carbohydrates: 26g

4.12 Turkey Meatballs
Preparation time: 10 Mins **Cooking time:** 30 Mins **Serving:** 4 Persons

Ingredients

- half cup fresh Parmesan cheese (grated)
- 1 pound ground turkey
- half cup fresh breadcrumbs (whole wheat)
- 2-3 tbsps of water
- 1 big egg (beaten)
- 1 tbsp fresh parsley (sliced)
- half tbsp fresh basil (sliced)
- half tbsp fresh oregano (sliced)
- Pinch of fresh nutmeg (grated)

Instructions

Get the oven ready at 350 degrees. Put parchment paper on two baking sheets. Mix the turkey, breadcrumbs, cheese, egg, water, herbs, nutmeg, salt, and pepper in a big container. Mix everything well. If the combination is too dry to form a ball, add a little more water. Roll the dough into 30 little balls. Put the balls in a neat row on the prepared baking sheets. Put in the oven and set the timer for 30 mins. To ensure even baking, flip the balls midway through the cooking time. Serve.

Nutrition Calories: 140 Kcal, Proteins: 14g, Fat: 9g, Carbohydrates: 5g

4.13 Chicken Chili and White Beans
Preparation time: 15 Mins **Cooking time:** 20 Mins **Serving:** 4 Persons

Ingredients

- 2 cups cooked chicken breast (shredded)
- 3 cups chicken stock

- 1 cup Brussels sprouts (sliced)
- 1 can (15-ounce) small white beans
- 1 cup nut milk
- 2 tbsps olive oil
- 1 leek (sliced)
- 1 tbsp ground cumin
- 1 small onion (sliced)
- 1 jalapeño pepper (seeded and diced)
- 2 garlic cloves (crushed)
- 1 tsp dried oregano
- Pinch of crushed red pepper flakes
- 1 big white potato (skinned and sliced)

Garnish:

- Tortilla chips
- Jalapeño slices
- Shredded cheese
- Hot sauce

Instructions

Put the olive oil in a saucepan and heat it over moderate heat. The onion, jalapeno, and the leak should be sautéed for around 5 mins. Mix in the garlic and seasonings. Prepare for one min. Include the chicken, stock, white beans, Brussels sprouts, and potatoes. Stir. Cover and cook at a low simmer for twenty mins. Don't forget the milk! Stir. Prepare for one min. Put on the garnishes and serve.

Nutrition Calories: 502 Kcal, Proteins: 45g, Fat: 12g, Carbohydrates: 58g

4.14 Cauliflower Rice and Salmon Container
Preparation time: 15 Mins **Cooking time:** 20 Mins **Serving:** 4 Persons

Ingredients

- half head cauliflower (riced)
- 2 salmon fillets
- 1 bunch kale (shredded)
- 1 tsp curry powder
- 3 tbsps olive oil
- 12 Brussels sprouts (halved)
- Himalayan salt

Marinade:

- 1 tbsp sesame seeds
- quarter cup tamari sauce

- 1 tsp Dijon mustard
- 1 tsp sesame oil
- 1 tsp maple syrup

Instructions

Get the oven ready at 350 degrees. Prepare parchment paper on a baking pan. The Brussels sprouts should be placed on the prepared baking sheet. Put a spoonful of olive oil on it and coat it well. Prepare by adding salt. Cook at 400° for 20 mins. Mix the marinade's components in a basin. Mix everything well. Substitute the salmon fillets for the Brussels sprouts on the baking pan. Drizzle the marinade over the fillets. Put in the oven for 15 mins. Place a tsp of olive oil in a saucepan and heat it over moderate heat. For three mins, sauté the kale. Put aside for the time being. Turn the heat to moderate and add the rest of the olive oil to the same pan. The curry powder, cauliflower rice, and salt should be added now. Stir-fry for three mins. Split the salmon and Brussels sprouts between two plates. To finish, drizzle some kale and cauliflower rice over the top. Serve.

Nutrition Calories: 502 Kcal, Proteins: 45g, Fat: 12g, Carbohydrates: 58g

4.15 Harissa and Chicken Tsideers

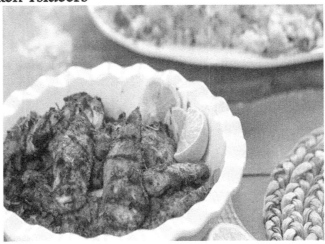

Preparation time: 15 Mins **Cooking time:** 15 Mins **Serving:** 6 Persons

Ingredients

- quarter cup plain Greek yogurt
- 2 tbsps harissa paste
- 24 pieces of chicken tsideers
- quarter cup dry white wine

Instructions

Place the yogurt, wine, and harissa in a container. Mix everything well. Chicken tenders should be inserted. Apply the marinade to the tsideers. Cover. Put the marinade into the fridge and let it sit for at least two hrs. Grills should be warm uped. The chicken strips need to be drained. Allow any surplus liquid to drain. Cook the tsideers on the grill for 5 mins total. You may make a sandwich out of the tenders. Add your favorite fresh herbs and sliced vegetables on top.

Nutrition Calories: 800 Kcal, Proteins: 51g, Fat: 37g, Carbohydrates: 62g

4.16 Chinese Chicken Salad
Preparation time: 15 Mins **Cooking time:** 10 Mins **Serving:** 4 Persons

Ingredients

Dressing:

- quarter-inch ginger (skinned and sliced)
- half cup vegetable oil
- quarter cup rice wine vinegar (unseasoned)
- 1 tbsp Dijon mustard
- 1 tbsp soy sauce (low-sodium)
- 2 garlic cloves (crushed)
- Pinch of salt
- 1 tsp sesame oil

Salad:

- quarter cup cooked edamame
- 4 cups green cabbage (shredded)
- 1 cup red cabbage (shredded)
- 2 cooked chicken breasts (shredded)
- half cup cilantro leaves (sliced)
- 1 small carrot (thin strips)
- 2 tbsps mint leaves (sliced)
- 4 scallions (thinly sliced)
- Wonton strips

Instructions

All the dressing components should be placed in a mixer and mixed together. Mix in a mixer and mix till smooth. Put everything that will go into the salad into a big mixing container. Dress the salad and serve. Put everything in a container and shake it up. Add wonton strips as a garnish. Serve.

Nutrition Calories: 97 Kcal, Proteins: 8.2g, Fat: 3g, Carbohydrates: 9g

4.17 Baked Cauliflower Buffalo
Preparation time: 15 Mins **Cooking time:** 10 Mins **Serving:** 4 Persons

Ingredients

- quarter cup water
- half cup hot sauce
- quarter cup banana flour
- 2 tbsps butter (melted)
- 1 moderate cauliflower (bite-sized)
- Pinch of pepper

- Ranch dressing (for serving)
- Pinch of salt

Instructions

First, set the oven temperature to 425 degrees F. Cover a baking tray with foil. Water, pepper, flour, and salt should be mixd in a container. Mix everything well. Cauliflower should be included. Mix well by tossing. Arrange the covered cauliflower in an even layer on the prepared baking sheet. Put in the oven for fifteen min. Midway during cooking time, turn the cauliflower over. The butter and spicy sauce should be mixd in a separate container. Mix everything well. Coat the cauliflower with the sauce. Add another 20 mins of baking time. Toss with ranch dressing and serve.

Nutrition Calories: 52 Kcal, Proteins: 2g, Fat: 2g, Carbohydrates: 6.4g

4.18 Kale and Sweet Potato Tostadas

Preparation time: 15 Mins **Cooking time:** 10 Mins **Serving:** 4 Persons

Ingredients

- 2 moderate sweet potatoes (cleaned and sliced)
- 8 stems of kale (roughly sliced)
- 12 Brussels sprouts (finely sliced)
- 1 tbsp lime juice
- 2 tbsps olive oil
- 1 tbsp olive oil
- Pinch of salt
- 1 tsp honey
- Corn tortillas
- Pinch of cayenne pepper
- Toasted coconut
- Fresh mint (sliced)
- Yogurt

Instructions

Turn the oven temperature up to 400 degrees F. Using foil, effective style baking sheets. The sweet potatoes should be placed on a baking pan that has been lined. Use olive oil as a finishing touch. Spike it up with some cayenne pepper. Just toss it on the coat. The greens should go on the second baking sheet that has been prepared in the same way. Dress with a drizzle of olive oil. Prepare by adding salt. Just toss it on the coat. Fire up the oven with both baking trays inside. For just around 10 mins, the kale may be roasted. For Forty mins, roast the sweet potatoes. Mix the Brussels sprouts, honey, and lime juice in a container. Mix well by tossing. Corn tortillas may be piled high on a sheet of aluminum foil. Put it in a warm uped 3-minute toasting cycle in the oven. Wrap the sweet potato and greens in a tortilla. Drizzle some toasted coconut, mint, yogurt, and Brussels sprouts on top. Serve.

Nutrition Calories: 190 Kcal, Proteins: 5g, Fat: 8g, Carbohydrates: 25g

CHAPTER 5: Anti-Inflammatory Snack Recipes

5.1 Spicy Tuna Rolls

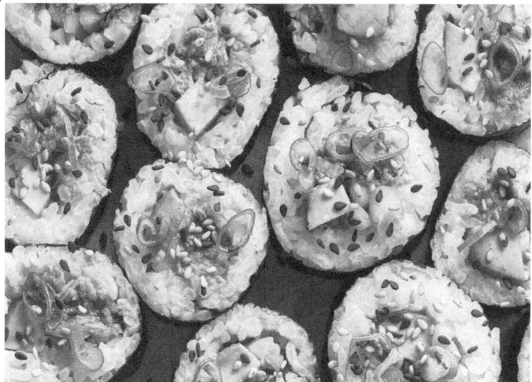

Preparation time: 15 Mins **Cooking time:** 10 Mins **Serving:** 4 Persons

Ingredients

- 1 moderate cucumber
- 1 pouch Yellowfin Tuna
- 1/16 tsp ground cayenne
- 2 avocado slices (cut into 6 pieces in total)
- one-eighth tsp pepper
- 1 tsp hot sauce
- one-eighth tsp salt

Instructions

Cut the cucumber into thin, long slices. Cucumbers used for slicing must be seedless. Generate a total of six servings. Roll the slices in paper towels to dry them. Mix the tuna, pepper, cayenne, salt, and spicy sauce in a container. Mix everything well. Top the cucumber rounds with the tuna spread. Avoid crowding the edges. The dish would benefit from one avocado slice. Carefully roll the cucumber. Insert toothpicks into each roll to keep it together. Serve.

Nutrition Calories: 190 Kcal, Proteins: 6g, Fat: 6g, Carbohydrates: 24g

5.2 Turmeric Gummies

Preparation time: 15 Mins **Cooking time:** 20 Mins **Serving:** 6 Persons

Ingredients

- 8 tbsps gelatin powder (unflavored)
- 3 half cups of water
- 6 tbsps maple syrup
- Pinch of ground pepper
- 1 tsp ground turmeric

Instructions

Mix the water, turmeric, and maple syrup in a saucepan and boil over moderate. Stir constantly and let cook for 5 mins. Shut off the furnace. Mix with some gelatin powder. Mix everything well. Bring the temperature up to maximum. In order to mix the gelatin powder, stir the contents of the saucepan vigorously. Fill molds made of silicon with the mixture. Cover. Put in the refrigerator and chill for at least four hrs. Cut them up into manageable gummy chunks. Serve.

Nutrition Calories: 22 Kcal, Proteins: 0g, Fat: 0g, Carbohydrates: 5.2g

5.3 Ginger-Cinnamon Mixed Nuts

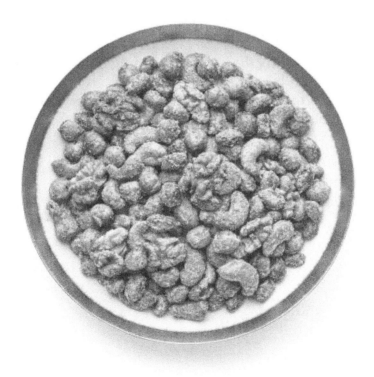

Preparation time: 10 Mins **Cooking time:** 15 Mins **Serving:** 4 Persons

Ingredients

- 2 big egg whites
- Coconut oil spray
- 2 cups mixed nuts

- 1 tsp fresh ginger (grated)
- half tsp fine sea salt
- half tsp ground Vietnamese cinnamon

Instructions

Get the oven ready at 250 degrees F. Place the egg whites in a big mixing dish. Mix with a mixer till foamy. Mix in the salt, ginger, and cinnamon. Mix all of the components by whipping them together. Add the roasted and salted mixed nuts. The coating may be achieved with a good mix. Spray coconut oil onto a sheet of parchment paper. Prepare a baking sheet with parchment paper. Create a flat layer of nuts on the baking sheet. Put it in the oven and set the timer for 40 mins. Halfway through, flip the baking sheet. It's best to wait till the nuts have cooled and hardened. Split them apart and use the pieces in various ways. Serve.

Nutrition Calories: 173 Kcal, Proteins: 5g, Fat: 16g, Carbohydrates: 6g

5.4 Ginger Date Almond Bars
Preparation time: 5 Mins **Cooking time:** 15 Mins **Serving:** 4 Persons

Ingredients

- 1 tsp ground ginger
- quarter cup almond milk
- 1 cup almond flour
- 3/4 cup dates

Instructions

Get the oven ready at 350 degrees. Mix the dates and almond milk in a mixer. Put everything in a mixer and whir it for 5 mins till it becomes a paste. Add the ground almonds and ginger. Put in other components and mix for three more mins. Place the components in a casserole. Hold off till it cools. Break up into eight bars. Serve.

Nutrition Calories: 270 Kcal, Proteins: 10g, Fat: 16g, Carbohydrates: 24g

5.5 Coffee Cacao Protein Bars
Preparation time: 5 Mins **Cooking time:** 20 Mins **Serving:** 8 Persons

Ingredients

- 18 big Medjool dates (pitted)
- 2 cups mixed nuts
- 1 cup egg white protein powder
- 3 tbsps instant coffee powder
- quarter cup cacao powder
- quarter cup cacao nibs
- 5 tbsps water

Instructions

Put parchment paper in an 8x8-inch square baking dish. Mix the coffee, egg white protein powder, cacao powder, and almonds in a mixing bowl. The nuts should be processed till they are in very minute bits. Include the dates. Combining procedure. Add water, 1 tbsp at a time, while processing, till a sticky consistency is reached. You need to take the processor's S-blade out.

Chop up the cacao nibs and add them to the mixture. Put the liquid into the prepared square baking dish. Use a roller to make the mixture uniformly flat. Keep cold for at least 60 mins. Separate into 16 pieces. Serve.

Nutrition

Calories: 246 Kcal, Proteins: 12g, Fat: 12g, Carbohydrates: 19g

Conclusion

The healthiest diet plan is probably that of a plant-based eater. Vegetarians and vegans are sometimes stereotyped as weak or sickly, especially by meat eaters and those with a preference for cheap cuisine. These are only two examples of the "legside issuances" that people who aren't acquainted with vegetarianism or vegetarian cookery believe exist. Most of the veggies and other natural items that tend to make up a vegetarian's or vegan's diet are really rather nutrient dense and calorie light. Superior nutrition and positive health benefits, such as the reduced risk of cancer, heart disease, and diabetes type 2, are provided by anti-inflammatory diets. Vegetarians and vegans weigh around 35 pounds less than meat eaters, according to the second Adventist Health Study. It is crucial to know the truth and reject the falsehoods about the health advantages of eating foods that originate from the soil. There really are great advantages to consuming food that originates from the soil.

Made in United States
Orlando, FL
08 July 2024

48719670R00070